How Dysfunctional Families Spur Mental Disorders

How Dysfunctional Families Spur Mental Disorders

A Balanced Approach to Resolve Problems and Reconcile Relationships

DAVID M. ALLEN, MD

Childhood in America
Sharna Olfman, Series Editor

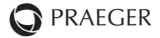 PRAEGER

AN IMPRINT OF ABC-CLIO, LLC
Santa Barbara, California • Denver, Colorado • Oxford, England

Library of Congress Cataloging-in-Publication Data

Allen, David M., 1949–
    How dysfunctional families spur mental disorders : a balanced approach to
resolve problems and reconcile relationships / David M. Allen.
        p. cm.—(Childhood in America)
    Includes bibliographical references and index.
    ISBN 978-0-313-39265-8 (hbk. : alk. paper)—ISBN 978-0-313-39266-5 (ebook)
1. Dysfunctional families—Psychological aspects. 2. Mental illness—Etiology.
3. Family psychotherapy. I. Title.
    RC455.4.F3A435   2010
    616.89′156—dc22   2010011250

ISBN: 978-0-313-39265-8
EISBN: 978-0-313-39266-5

14   13   12   11   10   1   2   3   4   5

This book is also available on the World Wide Web as an eBook.
Visit www.abc-clio.com for details.

Praeger
An Imprint of ABC-CLIO, LLC

ABC-CLIO, LLC
130 Cremona Drive, P.O. Box 1911
Santa Barbara, California 93116-1911

This book is printed on acid-free paper ∞

Manufactured in the United States of America

Contents

Introduction

Over the last three decades, a confluence of various factors and interests has changed the face of mental health treatment in the United States in ways that have been extremely detrimental to the mental health of some patients. The rise of managed health care, the increased influence of large pharmaceutical companies (known collectively as *big pharma*), popular irritation with individuals who want to blame everyone but themselves for their own shortcomings, the desire for quick fixes for complicated problems, the discovery that some mental illnesses actually are brain diseases and are not due to character flaws or bad mothering, the rise of neuroimaging technologies, and collective guilt stemming from major changes in child-rearing practices due to economic and social forces have all come together in a perfect storm.

The emphasis of psychological and psychiatric treatment has been gradually moving away from long, hard work on helping patients to alter well-ingrained problematic behavior and to fix highly unsatisfying family relationships. In its place are drug treatments for what are essentially behavioral problems and ultra-short-term "solution-oriented" psychotherapies. Understandable reactions to dysfunctional or disturbed family interactions that often lead to crippling anxiety, depression, and problem behavior have in some circles been suddenly turned into neuropsychiatric "diseases" or a product of defective mental functioning.

Many clinicians have narrowed their focus so much that they now aim to merely reduce unpleasant symptoms instead of remedying the situations that create the symptoms in the first place. Doing only this is like using a painkiller to treat the pain an individual suffers as someone continually stabs him or her in the shoulder with a penknife. I guess the medication would help such a person to tolerate the aching with more equanimity, but I think it would be better to help the patient find a way to stop the person with the knife. Just treating the symptom is putting a Band-Aid on a cancer.

ATTITUDES ABOUT FAMILY DYSFUNCTION

Family therapy, and the various theories and treatments that are called *family systems,* have taken an especially hard hit. These theories all share the view that dysfunctional interactions in families are the primary culprit in leading to many different psychological symptoms in individuals. In the 1980s and early 1990s, the extent of child abuse in this country and its high prevalence in the backgrounds of individuals with certain mental disorders became apparent in studies that were replicated many times. The terms *dysfunctional family* and *childhood sexual abuse* became a part of the common lexicon.

Family therapy and family systems theory were hot. A whole new tier of talk therapists arose to compete with psychiatrists, psychologists, and clinical social workers. Marriage and family counselors (MFCs)—later changing their name to marriage and family therapists (MFTs)—had their own schools and their own license and licensure examination in many states.

Gradually, however, due to a variety of factors that will be discussed in this book, family systems views began to lose favor, and people tired of what was framed the "abuse excuse" for bad behavior. The popular magazine for family therapists, *The Family Therapy Networker,* even changed its name to the *Psychotherapy Networker.* The psychotherapy field has always had fads in which new techniques were hailed as cure-alls and then suddenly disappeared, some never to be heard from again. Was family systems therapy just another one of these?

This book is a reexamination of some of the issues and excesses on all sides of the various debates, as well as the scientific, economic, and political forces that have, in my view, begun to lead the mental health field in the United States astray. As we shall see, part of the reason for this development is not just the reluctance of individuals to look at their own effect on other family members, but also because of the fact that, despite appearances to the contrary, people are also very protective of their immediate families. Rather than look at problematic behavior within the family, they would much rather blame their problems on mental deficits, miswired brains, or toxins in the environment like pesticides or sugary foods.

CAVEATS

Not all psychiatric diagnoses are creations of a psychiatric-industrial complex, and of course biological and genetic factors operate on all normal behavior and can make problematic reactions both more likely to occur and more likely to trigger later changes in brain functioning. As psychiatrist Leon Eisenberg pointed out,[1] "problems in living" and "diseases of the brain" are overlapping categories. In fact, I believe that the majority of psychiatric diagnoses are quite valid, and that biogenetic factors influence all behavior, even behavior that is seen only when individuals act in concert with others in a group. The diagnostic Bible of the profession, the *Diagnostic and Statistical Manual of Mental Disorders* (DSM),[2] has much that is admirable. I do, however, believe that the use of certain diagnoses has been taken to extreme, absurd, and dangerous heights.

This book will focus primarily on the treatment of relatively higher-functioning psychiatric and psychotherapy patients who carry psychiatric diagnoses such as personality disorders, anxiety disorders, and mood disorders. Although the subject of the severely and persistently mentally ill, such as individuals with chronic schizophrenia or autism, will be discussed, I will not be spending as much time on it. We now know that these are true brain diseases. The shameful way in which our society has abandoned the treatment and rehabilitation of these chronically impaired individuals to the streets and jails of America warrants its own whole book, and much has already been written on this subject.

Additionally, I will *not* be arguing, as some have, that psychopharmacology (use of medicines that alter processes within the central nervous system) and the variety of psychotherapy paradigms that are being used today are ineffective even when used properly and for appropriate patients; far from it. This is not a hysterical screed from someone who hates his own field or from a scientologist who thinks psychiatry is evil because mental illness is actually caused by space aliens and volcano gods. Nor am I a follower of Thomas Ssazz, who believes that all forms of mental illness are a myth and that schizophrenia is a normal reaction to a crazy culture.

As a psychiatrist, I have seen psychiatric medications work absolute wonders. I also have seen radical behavioral changes for the better in patients in psychotherapy through the use of a wide variety of different techniques, many of which I have incorporated into my own paradigm[3-5] for treating individuals with self-destructive or self-defeating behavior patterns. I have helped many individuals to reconcile with family members with whom they had previously been warring or from whom they had been estranged. These are the most moving experiences I have had as a therapist.

Paradoxically, many of the trends in the field that I believe to be countertherapeutic as well as counterproductive interfere with the incorporation and productive use of all of the new scientific knowledge that has been flooding the field. The recent explosion of techniques in neuroscience has been nothing short of breathtaking, and scientists have begun to help us understand enigmas that have vexed the field for decades. Psychotherapy innovators have begun to integrate the various competing and dissonant points of view in that endeavor, the debates over which have for too long scarred the field. New therapy methods have demonstrated impressive efficacy in many good studies.

In this book, I will be discussing in detail a lot of what is, in my opinion, bad science. This does not mean that I believe that science is bad. Good science is still the best way to sort out the truth about just about everything. However, science can be manipulated by scientists, organizations, and businesses to suit their needs. It can be "spun" in the same way that a politician spins the truth for political purposes. Study designs can be poor, studies can be selectively cited so that contradictory studies are not disseminated or well known, incorrect conclusions from studies can be drawn, and the strength of findings can be exaggerated.

Scientists, like everyone else, may operate with ulterior motives. They can manipulate data in their search for fame, fortune, or academic prestige. Still, the existence of bad or manipulated science does not justify quackery from snake oil salesman with no credentials at all who are touting ludicrous cures based on implausible theories.

I do not think there is some vast, widespread conspiracy to bilk patients out of their money and subject them to toxic treatments. The people who spin facts do so for their own individual interests, and their interests often compete with the interests of others who want to twist these same facts in a completely different direction. However, when the interests of several influential constituencies and organizations happen to coincide, the whole field can be moved in wrong directions.

As in any field, there are bad psychiatrists and psychologists who do the wrong thing, but there are plenty of good ones who do the right thing. Furthermore, any effective treatment also has potential

and actual side effects. Some of the side effects can, in a certain percentage of patients, be worse that the condition that is being treated.
In using any treatment, relative benefits and risks must be considered
and balanced against one another in order for a patient and doctor to
make an informed choice about whether or not to undergo the
therapy.

All of the information needed for clinicians to make truly
informed decisions is out there, if only they would take the time to
look for it. Debates about the issues discussed in this book are frequently held in readily available publications and other venues that
are directed at practitioners in the field.

My aim with this volume is to try to help lay readers become
better educated, more knowledgeable, and discerning consumers
of and advocates for mental health services. I will also suggest ways
to understand human behavior that may help to counteract the
destructive forces that have driven recent negative trends.

What is missing from much of today's mental health field is bal-
ance. Just as some Americans have become polarized over "red"
and "blue" political ideologies, the so-called experts who argue for
many of the opposing points of view within the field too frequently
go to extremes. When followed to their logical conclusions, some of
the ideas that they have advanced are frankly absurd. Thinking has
in many circles become either-or, black or white, you're with us or
you're against us. The type of thinking that has been called "both-
and" thinking, in which ideas that seem at first glance to be contradictory are found to be compatible through the understanding of
how the one idea relates to the other, has been in short supply. As
Eisenberg said, psychiatry and psychology do not have to be either
brainless (ignoring the physical reality of the central nervous system) or mindless (ignoring subjective human experience, emotion,
and cognition).

This book will also focus on the sociocultural forces that have
shaped the debate about who or what should be "blamed" by the
profession and by society for various psychological problems and
psychiatric disorders. In particular, what factors have led the role of
family interactions in both brain functioning and problematic individual behavior patterns to become marginalized?

Abbreviations

ABPN	American Board of Psychiatry and Neurology
ACGME	Accreditation Council for Graduate Medical Education
ADHD	attention deficit hyperactivity disorder
APA	American Psychiatric Association
BPD	borderline personality disorder
CBT	cognitive behavior therapy
CME	continuing medical education
CRO	contract research organization
DEA	Drug Enforcement Administration
DINKS	double income, no kids
DSM	*Diagnostic and Statistical Manual of Mental Disorders*
DTC	direct to consumer advertising
ERISA	Employee Retirement Income Security Act of 1974
FDA	Food and Drug Administration
FMRI	functional magnetic resonance imaging
FMSF	False Memory Syndrome Foundation
IOM	Institute of Medicine
MFCC	marriage, family, and child counselor
MFT	marriage and family therapist
NAMI	National Alliance on Mental Illness
NCANDS	National Child Abuse and Neglect Data System
NEA-BPD	National Education Alliance for Borderline Personality Disorder
NIDA	National Institute on Drug Abuse
NIH	National Institutes of Health

NIMH	National Institute of Mental Health
NMS	neuroleptic malignant syndrome
NOS	not otherwise specified
PhRMA	Pharmaceutical Research and Manufacturers of America
RCT	randomized clinical trial
RRC	residency review committee
SEPI	Society for the Exploration of Psychotherapy Integration
SIB	self-injurious behavior
SSRI	selective serotonin reuptake inhibitor
TAU	treatment as usual
YAVIS	young, attractive, verbal, intelligent, and successful

1

The Brainlessness-
Mindlessness Pendulum

A good place to start is the broad swings of Eisenberg's brainlessness-mindlessness pendulum in the history of American psychiatry (mental health treatment as practiced by physicians) over the last century or so. I will show in particular how differing ideas about morality have affected an ongoing debate about whether biological or environmental factors, especially the influence of other people in the environment, are more important in causing mental problems.

Over the last century, psychiatry has moved wildly from thinking solely in terms of the brain to thinking solely in terms of the mind, and then back again to only the brain. At present, a hyperblown biogenetic disease model for all recurrent human behavior problems has gained relative prominence in psychiatric thinking. Of course, the breadth of opinion within the field has always been and remains quite wide due to the omnipresence of countervailing voices that speak against any predominant viewpoint.

The issue of who or what is responsible for various forms of human misbehavior and for everyday emotional misery is of course debated in the popular culture as much as it is by people within the mental health professions. We all have an interest in what makes people tick and especially in the causes of emotional problems. Since most psychiatric conditions have no obvious causative agent such as a microbe or a traumatic physical injury, the "nature-nurture" debate continues to rage in many different public arenas. (The current state of the science on this question will be discussed in detail in Chapter Five.) Much of what is said in these debates is influenced by commonly believed myths as well as by hidden personal or political agendas.

Both clinicians and researchers may bias their work because of pressure from prevailing cultural forces or because of their own idiosyncratic views about what is moral and what is not. They read about and are influenced by public opinion, even as they belittle it as nothing more than the ideas of untrained laypeople who have no expertise in psychology. Their political, social, and religious passions may make certain cultural viewpoints more appealing to them than others.

A second source of cultural pressures on clinicians to champion certain points of view stems from the fact that they are in business to sell their services. If a significant number of potential clients boycott their practices because of their reputation for "blaming the victim," "parent bashing," or "undermedicating," then they suffer financially. Researchers, on the other hand, may need the support of opinionated public advocacy groups like the National Alliance on Mental Illness (NAMI) to help finance and disseminate their findings, thereby helping their academic careers.

In the next section, I briefly discuss how theories about which human characteristics are inherited genetically gave rise to a vicious and twisted ideology that led to the systematic murder of millions of people. After the full results of the application of this ideology became widely known and appreciated, any discussion about biological inheritance of human traits became an anathema in much of psychiatry.

EUGENICS

In the late nineteenth and early twentieth century, the medical community assumed that the ultimate etiology of all mental illnesses was *organic* (physical). Even Sigmund Freud, the originator of medical psychotherapy or talk therapy, had originally hoped to better understand the biological foundations of mental phenomena. Unfortunately, the technology to do so did not exist. Even severe mental illnesses such as schizophrenia and manic-depressive illness were at that time completely impervious to any type of laboratory investigation.

The Austrian monk Gregor Mendel discovered in the mid-1800s that certain physical characteristics of plants and animals were passed down from one generation to the next and that the way that traits were expressed in each generation seemed to follow certain rules. Although scientists did not know anything about the physical structure of genes or the biological mechanisms through which they operated for quite some time afterwards, they were curious about which human characteristics might follow Mendelian genetic laws. They began to study human pedigrees: family trees showing which members of extended families over several generations exhibited certain traits. Mental retardation and mental illnesses were of particular interest, even though Mendelian genetic laws had only been shown to be true for the inheritance of some physical attributes.

The biological underpinnings of many mental phenomena clearly have their origin in genetics. Although they are hardly the only determinants of brain functioning, our genes set the parameters by which the structure and abilities of the human brain develop and change over the lifespan. The subtleties of how the brain functions and what behavioral attributes have genetic components are only now beginning to become clear, but despite the lack of knowledge in earlier times, an interest in the inheritance of mental characteristics was certainly understandable.

In the 1880s, a cousin of Charles Darwin named Francis Galton began to think about the relationship between Mendelian genetics and the theory of natural selection in evolution. The idea that the forces of nature seem to favor the strongest and most adaptive creatures led him to formulate a social philosophy that he called *eugenics*. He believed that the human race could be improved if society would select which individuals would be allowed or not be allowed to have children, based on what he believed to be their biologically inherited characteristics. The list of presumed inherited characteristics was, even by the loose standards of some of today's "biological" psychiatrists, absurdly broad. Characteristics thought by many followers of eugenics to be genetically transmitted included such traits as sexual promiscuity and even poverty.

Eugenics quickly found many prominent believers, particularly in Germany and the United States. Among them were Luther Burbank, Alexander Graham Bell, feminist icon Margaret Sanger, the Carnegie Institute, and the Ford and Rockefeller Foundations. The philosophy gradually expanded from an emphasis on selective breeding or positive eugenics to the idea that "inferior" members of our species should be forcibly sterilized so that they would never be able to pass down their supposedly bad characteristics. This was termed negative eugenics. Some people who believed that forced sterilization was a moral endeavor eventually jumped to the idea that inferior peoples should be exterminated.

In the United States, the influx of large numbers of European immigrants led to fears that such people might be of inferior stock and might therefore "pollute" or "contaminate" the gene pool. Because eugenics gave voice and legitimacy to these fears, it was appealing to a large segment of the American population. In 1910, a man named Harry H. Laughton established an organization called the Eugenics Record Office (ERO), through which he lobbied politicians to help protect the purity of the human race through restrictions on immigration of peoples from southern and eastern Europe. The peoples from these regions were thought to have "excessive insanity." The efforts of the organization led to the passage of the 1924 Johnson-Reed immigration bill, which successfully limited the immigration of people from these areas and completely excluded Asians from entering the United States.

The ERO also advocated forced sterilizations of certain segments of society. It was supported financially by the Carnegie Institute, among others. The idea of forced sterilization of the mentally retarded had already gained acceptance by the time of the ERO's founding, and the first state law requiring it was passed in Indiana in 1907. Eventually, thirty states passed similar laws, resulting in the forced sterilization of over 60,000 Americans. The practice did not completely stop until approximately 1963.

Laughton was unhappy with the earliest versions of state laws mandating this practice and with their lax enforcement. He also felt that forced sterilizations should include not just the "feebleminded" but also the insane, criminals, epileptics, alcoholics, and even the deaf and blind. He apparently believed that all of these characteristics were inherited through genetic mechanisms and that any chance of their being passed on to children had to be eliminated. He drafted a model law in 1922 that became a template for some later state laws.

Laughton was also influential in a case that came to the United States Supreme Court in which the constitutionality of the forced sterilization of the mentally retarded was upheld: the case of *Buck v. Bell* in 1927. Carrie Bell was a woman who was branded as being mentally retarded after she became pregnant following a rape by the nephew of her foster parents. She was very likely of normal intelligence, as was her daughter Vivian. Nonetheless, no less a figure than Justice Oliver Wendell Holmes led the way in ruling in favor of the state of Virginia, writing, "Three generations of imbeciles are enough."

Adolph Hitler and his henchmen found this ruling by an American court inspiring. They loosely used Laughlin's model law in drafting Germany's own "Law for the Prevention of Genetically Diseased Offspring," which went into effect in 1934. In 1936, Laughlin was granted an honorary degree from the University of Heidelberg in Germany for his work on behalf of "racial cleansing." In a sublime irony, Laughlin himself developed epilepsy in his later years. Sufferers of this disorder were some of the people he thought should be eliminated from the planet.

The mentally retarded, followed in quick succession by the mentally ill, were among the first victims of the Nazi death machine. Forced sterilizations began in 1935, followed by the T-4 program for "euthanasia" of the mentally ill in 1939. One of the architects of this death program was a psychiatrist, Ernst Rudin, as were several of the doctors directly involved in it. The methods he helped devise for killing individuals with mental problems were later adapted for use in the large-scale attempted extermination of those ethnic groups that the Nazis considered genetically inferior, such as the Jews and the Gypsies, as well as of certain individuals within their own ethnic group such as homosexuals.

In the early days of the T-4 program, even small children were not spared. At one point some families of children with mental problems, who were being told that their offspring had died peacefully of natural causes, became suspicious because they learned that so many of their children seemed to have all died on the same days. To keep the program secret, the Nazis stopped killing the children directly in favor of just letting them starve to death so they would all die on different days.

Meanwhile, back in the United States, support for eugenics waned by the end of the 1930s because of its association with the Nazis and also because the so-called science behind it was proving to be quite poor. The Carnegie Institute withdrew its funding of the ERO in 1935, and it soon folded. Some psychiatrists in the United States, however, apparently did not get the message.

A psychiatrist named Foster Kennedy gave an address to the American Psychiatric Association's annual meeting in 1941. In it, he strongly advocated not only the forcible sterilization of the mentally retarded but also their extermination, especially if they fell below a certain functional level. Because he assumed that such individuals were in constant suffering and would be better off dead, he referred to this killing as euthanasia or mercy killing. His address was published in the *Journal of the American Psychiatric Association* in July of 1942.[1] In the same issue an opposing viewpoint by another psychiatrist, Leo Kanner, was also published,[2] along with an editorial.[3]

While Kanner had no objection to sterilization, he did object to euthanasia. He also questioned the validity of assuming that people of low IQ would necessarily beget children who were also mentally deficient, but he did not spend any time exploring the ramifications that would ensue for his philosophy if this were indeed the case. He believed that sterilization should be reserved only for those who could not perform useful work. He feared that stopping more functional people of low intelligence from reproducing might lead to a labor shortage in unskilled occupations, which would adversely affect the functioning of society. Of note is the fact that, by July of 1942, psychiatrists were already aware of what was going on in Germany. Kanner noted, "If [journalist and historian] William Shirer's report is true—and there are reasons to believe that it is true—in Nazi Germany the Gestapo is now systematically bumping off the mentally deficient people of the Reich" (p. 21).

The *Journal*'s editorial on the debate foreshadowed the sea change that was about to take place in psychiatric thinking. The writers agreed that, if euthanasia should be allowed, it should be reserved for only the most hopeless and nonfunctional individuals. They also thought that the reactions of the parents should be an important consideration. However, they raised the possibility that if a family had "unwholesome" relationships, they might have contributed to the development their child's "illness."

In other words, they thought that disturbed parents could cause at least some cases of extremely low intelligence. The editors also strongly implied that any parents who were worth their salt would welcome the relief provided by the euthanasia of their child and would understand that their child should be put out of its misery for its own good. Any parents who opposed such mercy killing were possibly victims of "exaggerated sentimentality and forced devotion" motivated by morbid guilt. Such parents were probably in need of treatment designed to free them of the "unhappy obsession of obligation or guilt" (p. 143). This was one early example of the trend toward blaming parental behavior for what are essentially physical and not psychological disorders in their children.

PSYCHOANALYSIS

Collective horror at the revelations of the Holocaust after World War II made eugenics as well as any other genetic explanations for human behavior taboo for a large segment of American society. The combination of this cultural attitude and the lack of scientific technology for studying the brain and its functions made psychiatry rife for takeover by philosophies that were based more on humanism than on hard science. In particular, psychiatrists who were already by this time fans of Sigmund Freud became far more influential in the field.

Freud's theories looked to the environment, in particular the social and family environment, and to the inner workings of human consciousness to explain problematic behavioral syndromes. This shift away from biology and genetics occurred in the United States despite the fact that the majority of individuals in this country still thought that African Americans and other foreign peoples were genetically and intellectually inferior.

Freud's theory of psychoanalysis explained human problem behavior and emotions by looking at the influence of early family experiences on the psychological development of young children. Briefly, all young children were believed to be born uncivilized. Proper parenting was believed to be required to help children successfully learn to channel their many wild biological urges and drives into socially appropriate avenues. According to the analysts, if the parents had emotional problems themselves, this learning process in their children might be thwarted. This in turn would lead to an unresolved conflict in the child's mind between certain bodily urges (the *id*) and the values he or she had learned through family experiences (the *superego* or conscience).

Because this *intrapsychic conflict* produced anxiety for the thinking part of the mind (the *ego*), the conflict as well as the memories behind it would be *repressed* into an *unconscious* part of the mind, where they would continue to adversely affect the child's behavior as he or she grew into adulthood. Intrapsychic conflict was felt by dogmatic analysts to be the cause of almost all psychological disturbances and disorders. Therapy consisted of talking to patients in ways that would help them uncover these unconscious infantile experiences so that they would no longer be controlled by them. This treatment became known informally as talk therapy or psychotherapy.

Psychoanalysis had already started to gain prominence in the United States in the 1920s. Sigmund Freud, a Jew from Vienna, and many of his most influential followers were forced to flee Austria when the Nazis came to power. Many of his disciples came to the United States. After the war, several different psychoanalytically oriented theories and therapies combined to become the dominant approach in much of American psychiatry. This happened despite the fact that psychoanalysis was rejected as unscientific by most mainstream researchers in nonmedical academic psychology departments across the country. Psychoanalysis was developed and taught in independent, insular *institutes*, within which academic and scientific rigor was sometimes lacking.

Even severe mental illnesses like schizophrenia, though known even then to be completely unresponsive to psychoanalytic therapy, were thought by analysts to have their causal roots in the effect of the early family environment on childhood development. The term *neurosis*, which means maladaptive behavior based on conflicts within an individual's mind between bodily urges and conscience, was part of the name of many psychiatric diagnoses in the first two editions of the *Diagnostic and Statistical Manual of Mental Illness* (DSM). Although analysts gave lip service to the idea that genetic or constitutional factors played a part in mental illness, psychoanalysts focused almost exclusively on the workings of the mind and not of the brain.

From the late 1920s until the late 1950s, much of the cultural life in the United States was heavily influenced by psychoanalytic ideas. Analytic notions became incorporated into the common discourse, and to this day they remain part of our usual understanding of much of human behavior. Many people use analytic ideas all the time without knowing that they are doing so. Concepts such as "arrested development" and "inferiority complex" are common parlance. The Freudian *defense mechanisms* are invoked to explain a wide range of behavioral phenomena. For example, people who are angry at certain individuals but cannot stand up to them are commonly said to "take their anger out on someone else." This is an example of the defense mechanism known as *displacement*.

According to Eisenberg,[4] in the early 1960s more than half of the chairmen of medical school psychiatry departments were members of analytic societies. In 1962 at an American Psychiatric Association conference on education in psychiatry, Eisenberg was practically ridden out of town on a rail for suggesting that rigid analytic orthodoxy might have started to become a conceptual barrier to further progress in the field.

Nonetheless, as early as the 1950s, the pendulum swing to a brainless phase of psychiatry began to lose some steam, and it was ever so gradually nudged in the other direction. That decade saw the discovery almost through sheer accident of three new classes of medications that had powerful and highly beneficial effects on severe mental illnesses: phenothiazine antipsychotics for schizophrenia, tricyclic antidepressants for clinical depression, and lithium for manic-depressive illness, now called bipolar disorder.

The dramatic response of these conditions to medication, coupled with their imperviousness to psychoanalytic treatment, emboldened those psychiatrists and neuroscientists who still believed that these disorders were due to pathological changes in the brain rather than to mental complexes. If in fact these three disorders were primarily bio-genetic in origin, many reasoned, other psychiatric disorders must also be caused primarily by brain pathology.

BIOLOGICAL PSYCHIATRY

A few years later, the advent of the placebo-controlled clinical trial, to be described later, provided a means to scientifically assess the effectiveness of different treatments. So-called biological psychia-try was born, and it began to take over American psychiatry. The field moved from the brainlessness of the "pure" psychoanalysts back to the mindlessness of the "pure" neurobehaviorists. Biology became destiny, and the role of genetics was restored to its former lofty position. At least in psychiatry if not in the other mental health disciplines, mindlessness has now gotten completely out of hand, as we shall see, with its proponents using a disease model to explain some very normal human feelings and behavior.

Talk of genetic differences and abnormalities still can raise hackles, however. Earlier in the twentieth century, when academic psychologists began looking at differences in average intelligence in various racial and ethnic groups, particularly in blacks, they opened a hornet's nest. The controversy continues to rage, although speak-ing of it has become somewhat politically incorrect. Whenever com-parisons are made, blacks on average score lower on IQ tests than Anglo whites.

Of course, some black people score much higher on the tests than most whites, while some whites score much lower than most blacks. (This phenomenon of a wide *scatter* between different scores in different populations on psychological and medical tests is commonplace.) The scatter of IQ scores did not stop groups like the Ku Klux Klan, who advocated for continued racial segregation, from seizing on the original observation about IQs as an argument for the genetic inferiority of blacks. Somehow they also used this assertion to justify continuing to keep black people from economic and social advancement. By that reasoning, I guess members of Mensa should be allowed to enslave everyone else.

The debate was rekindled by the publication of the book *The Bell Curve*[5] by Richard Herrnstein and Charles Murray in 1996, which became a bestseller. Most forward-thinking people were under-standably outraged that the purveyors of racism seized on the book to again argue for black racial inferiority. However, even among these individuals, understanding the differences in performance on IQ tests between blacks and whites was still difficult.

The results of psychological tests can be very misleading. Perhaps the IQ test difference can be explained, not by racial differences, but by the fact that American black people might have a good reason to be unmotivated to do well on IQ tests and therefore not take them as seriously as do whites. No means currently exist to accurately assess test takers' motivation to do well, but such motivation certainly influences scores on tests.

As many African American commentators have pointed out, not all that long ago blacks who looked smart were called "uppity" and were in significant danger of being lynched. The comic Chris Rock tells a joke about a black motorist who stopped at a stop sign in the South and was therefore shot by a police officer because he had the ability to read the sign. The mechanism by which fears based on experiences like this might be transmitted from one generation to another despite cultural changes, while the original reasons for the fear become hidden, will be discussed in the next chapter.

THE ARROGANCE OF PSYCHOANALYSTS

The ascendancy of biological psychiatry was further abetted by the ongoing hubris of the psychoanalysts, who tried to explain everything under the sun using psychoanalytic theory and refused to subject the clinical outcomes of their treatments to scientific scrutiny. I personally encountered a dramatic example of this arrogance during my psychiatric training as a resident in the mid-1970s. In talking to other psychiatrists over the years, I know that my experience was not unique. At that time, most of the psychiatrists on my medical faculty were psychoanalysts. Analysts no longer say what I am about to relate, but many still maintain the beliefs that underlie the statement.

In order to fully understand what was said to me, one must first understand that analysts believe that ideas and feelings that are threatening to individuals because of an intrapsychic conflict are often *resisted* by them in a variety of different ways. Although this is often true, I found that when I questioned certain ideas within analytic theory, I was told that I needed to get into therapy to find out why I was resistant to these concepts.

The sheer audacity and scope of the faulty reasoning in this retort are breathtaking. If I were on a debate team, I would identify at least three different logical fallacies wrapped up in this one statement. First, it is a nonsequitur, which means the conclusion does not necessarily follow from the premise. I might be resisting the concept because I felt threatened by it, but I might also be questioning it for some other reason. Second, it is a personal or ad hominem attack on me rather than an argument about the validity of my questions. Third and most serious, it begs the question. It presumes that psychoanalytic theory is correct, when that is precisely what I was calling into question.

Another example of analytic arrogance is psychoanalysts' refusal to do outcome studies on the effectiveness of psychoanalytic therapy. Their justification for this was a version of the Heisenberg Uncertainty Principle in physics. This principle states that many of the characteristics of an entity under study, such as a subatomic particle, cannot be completely known to scientists because the mere act of looking at them changes them from what they were before. For instance, if a physicist uses light to measure the behavior of a subatomic particle, the energy of the light used slightly changes the particle's behavior or its position in space.

Psychoanalysis is theorized to work through the analysis of something called *transference*, a phenomenon in which a person reacts to another person as if he or she were a parent or some other early attachment figure. If a patient had difficulty with, say, an authoritarian father, he might react to anyone in a position of authority in the same way that he reacted to his father in the past. Psychoanalysts used to think that, because they revealed nothing about themselves or what they really thought during psychotherapy, they therefore could become "blank screens" on which patients would "project" these transference feelings. The transference could then be analyzed in the ongoing relationship between the patient and therapist in the here and now.

The analysts reasoned that if a third party such as a researcher were to talk to either the patient or the analyst during therapy, the transference would be "contaminated." This supposedly changed the treatment immutably, probably for the worse, and therefore the research would not be valid anyway.

Of course, a therapist cannot really be a completely blank screen. The patient can discern many things about the "real" therapist just by the way he or she decorates the office or shifts uncomfortably in a chair when the patient brings up a specific topic. Most of today's analysts are no longer dogmatic on this issue and are now willing to do at least some outcome studies.

Another facet of the psychoanalysts' arrogance that had a most dramatic effect on the ambient culture, which in turn boomeranged on the field, was that they had a tendency to use theories about family behavior as a substitute for actual observations of families behaving. In no area was this conduct more outrageous than in psychoanalytic ideas about two psychiatric conditions that are now well accepted by almost all mental health professionals to be actual brain diseases: schizophrenia and infantile autism (previously called childhood schizophrenia). In the next chapter, I discuss what transpired in this regard as well as some cultural events that have led to the mental health field's deemphasis on dysfunctional family interaction as a major risk factor for any and all behavioral problems in favor of a disease model.

2

Don't Blame Us

Michael Kerr, a protégé of the late family therapy pioneer Murray Bowen, lectures about something he calls the "reality wagon" and how easy it is to fall off the wagon. On one side of the reality wagon is the belief "It is all my fault." On the other side is the belief "I had nothing to do with it." In a modern free society, anyone taking either extreme position when discussing what ultimately happens in his or her life is often, though not always, living in Fantasyland. While much of what happens to us is beyond our control, we are all to some degree the authors of our own lives. How we react and cope with what life throws at us plays a large role in where we end up. Misplaced blame and inappropriate guilt interfere with attempts to solve problems in living and problems in relationships. Both lead to bad feelings and interpersonal conflict.

In discussing the origins of various mental disorders, the issues of blame and guilt have had a particularly malignant effect because the determination of which disorders are true brain diseases, which stem primarily from psychological and interpersonal problems, and which stem from a combination of both remains unsettled for many of them. This chapter will examine the effects of blame and guilt in several different arenas within American society that have impacted the treatment of mental and behavioral disorders.

SCHIZOPHRENIA AND THE FAMILY

Although dysfunctional family interactions can be risk factors for worsening the symptoms of schizophrenia once the disorder is already present, they are clearly not risk factors for its initial development. That the brains of these unfortunate individuals perform very abnormally is a virtual certainty, despite the fact that after decades of effort by neuroscientists we have not been able to precisely pin down the nature of the organic problems in the disorder. This latter fact is often cited by critics of psychiatry as "proof" that schizophrenia is not a real disease.

This argument is weak because we do know that a major problem in the brains of schizophrenics is the nature of the network of connections between the millions of brain cells known as *synapses*, and we are not even close to fully understanding how neural networks are formed or function in the *normal* human brain. Our knowledge of how different genes and environmental influences combine to determine which nerve cells connect with which others is in its infancy. Such knowledge is essential to fully understand pathological neural networks.

In the past when we knew even less about brain functioning than we do today, schizophrenia was theorized by psychoanalysts to be a *functional* or psychological disorder created by a *schizophrenogenic mother*. Without going into details, the purported schizophrenogenic mother was thought to literally drive her child crazy. This idea was in no way based on actual observation of the way members of the families of schizophrenics interacted with one another, but was based purely on psychoanalytic theories of the mind.

Psychoanalysts were later joined in blaming schizophrenia on dysfunctional family interactions by a group of therapists known as family systems therapists. Their explanations for deviant human behavior are quite different from those of the analysts, and as we will see in later chapters, many of their theories are quite powerful. However, they unfortunately undermined their own credibility by concocting explanations for schizophrenia that also seemed to pin the blame for the delusions and hallucinations of these patients on parents.

Some family therapists could at least claim that, unlike the analysts, they had observed the families of schizophrenics in action. When family systems originators first tried to study family behavior under controlled conditions, the easiest families for them to sequester and then observe were those of the schizophrenic patients who were institutionalized. The initial observations of these families led to the *double bind* theory of schizophrenia.

This theory posited that schizophrenia was caused by parents constantly subjecting their young ones to impossible-to-solve, no-win dilemmas. The parents would demand certain actions, but the children on whom the demands were placed would be damned if they followed instructions, and yet also damned if they did not. They were not allowed to comment on the bind they were placed in, and as children they were also not free to leave the family.

Double binding in families definitely does exist as an important characteristic of human behavior and, in my experience, has markedly untoward effects on its recipients. Mixed messages and poor communication skills are two of the defining and most important hallmarks of so-called dysfunctional families. The problem with the early family therapists applying this idea to schizophrenia was that they did not compare families of schizophrenics with families of patients with other types of emotional troubles. If they had, they would have seen that double binds were just as common if not more common in many families that do not produce a schizophrenic child as they are in those that do.

Double binds may also be one aspect of a family characteristic called *expressed emotion*, which is defined as high levels of anger and emotionality in the family as a whole. High expressed emotion has been shown in multiple studies to be a risk factor for acute exacerbations of the disorder in schizophrenic individuals who are already known to have the disorder. Families with high expressed emotion may have been overrepresented in hospital populations, since only the more disturbed patients with the disorder are hospitalized, leading family therapists to see it more frequently than they might have if they had included observations of families with schizophrenic members who were more stable.

CHILDHOOD AUTISM AND THE FAMILY

The history of theories about the origins of infantile autism in psychiatry is even more reprehensible and outrageous than that of schizophrenia. Even though once again we do not now know precisely how or why, we do know that the parts of the brain known to be responsible for social behavior and the reading of social cues are miswired in autistic children. In the 1950s and 1960s, a psychoanalyst name Bruno Bettelheim came up with the hare-brained idea that this condition, which is in all likelihood present from birth, is caused by so-called *refrigerator mothers*. This theory held that the mothers of autistic children were so cold, rigid, and intellectual that their babies became unresponsive to social interaction. Bettelheim appears to have based his theory both on earlier psychoanalytic writings and on the famous experiments of Harry Harlow with monkeys. Monkey babies taken from their mothers and raised in social isolation do not respond normally to other monkeys.

Rumors abound that Bettelheim faked his data to make it look stronger than it was. I highly doubt that he actually observed the interactions between autistic children and their mothers more than casually, but analysts spoke about his theories as if they were well-established facts. In a brief interaction, the mothers of autistic children may appear to be unresponsive, but that is because they have already learned through experience that trying to be responsive does not accomplish much with an autistic infant.

A version of this argument—that parents act in inappropriate ways only in response to the behavior of difficult, brain-disordered children—is commonly and inappropriately used to explain away the role of child abuse and neglect in a wide variety of psychological disorders. However, child mistreatment and the alleged unresponsive behavior of "refrigerator mothers" are only superficially analogous, as we shall see later.

Another good argument against Bettelheim's theory has also been misapplied to other disorders: Bettelheim ignored the probably telling fact that many of the mothers whom he labeled as inherently cold interacted very warmly with their spouses and with their other, nonautistic children. They were not human refrigerators as advertised.

Again, this reasoning was turned on its head when some people argued that, if siblings turn out differently from one another, the differences must be due solely to their genetics and not to family dysfunction. The problem with applying this reasoning to discrepancies in the way siblings turn out in other disorders is that parents do not treat all of their children even remotely the same. Bettelheim's formulation implied, in contrast, that coldness was a fundamental aspect of the personalities of mothers of autistic children, which should therefore affect many of their other relationships. This was clearly not the case.

As more and more good information came out about the clearly biological origins of both schizophrenia and infantile autism, a huge, righteous, and very understandable backlash against both psychoanalysts and family therapists developed among the parents of afflicted individuals. These parents became more and more outraged as time went on. How dare these so-called experts blame their children's illnesses on bad parenting? Mothers and fathers of the mentally ill began to organize in revolt. This was one factor in the formation and development of the National Alliance for the Mentally Ill (NAMI), an organization founded in 1979.

THE NATIONAL ALLIANCE FOR THE MENTALLY ILL

NAMI was primarily formed to fight for the proper treatment of the chronically mentally ill. Its rise was spurred by political developments that took place during the times that Ronald Reagan was governor of California and later president of the United States. As governor in the late 1960s and 1970s, Reagan presided over the emptying of taxpayer-supported state mental hospitals.

The impetus for taking this action was well intentioned. It was meant to be beneficial to both patients with chronic schizophrenia and taxpayers alike. Since the advent of antipsychotic medications, or so the reasoning went, warehousing these unfortunate human beings in institutions was no longer humane or necessary. With their psychosis under control, afflicted individuals could now have freer lives out among the rest of us and be treated for their illness as outpatients in Community Mental Health Centers. This idea spread like kudzu from California to the rest of the country.

A major problem with this plan arose because the Community Mental Health Centers were never adequately funded. Since the mentally ill rarely vote, money for their needs was often was often the first thing sacrificed during economic downturns. With a tax-cutting frenzy gripping the country for decades, tax money for this purpose continues to dry up even now, and mental health treatment for the seriously and persistently mentally ill has fallen to new lows. Chronic schizophrenics often are seen once or not at all at community centers following discharge from a hospital after an acute episode, and then lost to follow-up.

Since they are not getting the medication they need, this lack of follow-up sets up a revolving door in which they soon end up back in the hospital. With hospital beds also drying up, we now have a situation in which a larger number of severely mentally ill individuals are being treated in jails than in mental hospitals. The increasing problem with homelessness can also be directly attributed to these events, since a high percentage of the homeless are mentally ill patients who have not been taking their medication.

When the Reagan administration took over Washington in 1980, it began a program of purging chronic schizophrenics and other mentally ill patients from Social Security Disability (SSD) rolls. I saw firsthand the damage this caused. I was in private practice in southern California at the time and often performed psychiatric evaluations on patients filing for disability payments for Social Security. Suddenly patients dependent on disability payments were being reevaluated every single year, and both new and old applicants were being denied benefits. At times what I wrote about them in my psychiatric assessments did not seem to matter in the final determination of their disability status. Most of these applicants had severe and highly incapacitating mental problems. There was no way these people could hold a job. The administration's effort to purge the disability rolls was finally stopped by judges in federal courts.

NAMI has done an excellent job of fighting for the rights of the mentally ill, but some members have become overzealous about the unrelated issue of the role of parents in the behavior problems of their offspring. Their justifiable and completely understandable outrage at being blamed by therapists for causing autism and schizophrenia started to spread to their ideas about other psychological conditions and disorders. They began to advocate the position that, since dysfunctional family interactions do not cause some disorders, they therefore cannot be considered as potential causative factors for any mental problems at all. Bad parenting practices were seen as inconsequential; children were thought to turn out the way that they do because that is the way they were genetically programmed to be.

This argument is a bit like saying that because a "fossil" known as the "Piltdown Man" proved to be a fraud, that therefore paleontologists should ignore all fossil evidence. This type of logical fallacy is known as *overgeneralization* in a type of psychotherapy called cognitive therapy. It is frequently used in informal arguments and sometimes in academic presentations by people involved in mental health, even by those who should know better. Many times it is used disingenuously. Other examples of the tactic of using disingenuous arguments in scientific debates will be seen throughout this book.

Family systems theory posits that, in dysfunctional families, one family member is often scapegoated when in fact the interactions of everyone in the family are problematic. The scapegoated individual, usually one of the children, is then brought in by the family for treatment. For this reason, the scapegoat is called the *identified patient*, as opposed to the actual patient, the family. Since generally the parents within a family are considered to be far more powerful agents than are children, this formulation can easily be misinterpreted as blaming the parents, rather than the identified patient, for the emotional problems of a child, even after the child is grown.

Never mind that mental "conditions" such as personality disorders, the subject of Chapter Eight, are in no way analogous to conditions such as schizophrenia. Suddenly *any* recurrent behavioral problem could be considered a brain disease. Gradually, a significant portion of the population came to believe that it was politically incorrect to blame any family member for anything that happened

to any other member. Even the role of child abuse in the development of emotional problems was minimized, as I shall discuss in
detail in the next chapter. Family systems therapy became one of
NAMI's public enemies. Parent advocacy groups for different disorders, patterned after NAMI, began to show up at professional
meetings such as the annual meeting of the American Psychiatric
Association (APA), ready to pounce on any speaker who seemed to
violate this new orthodoxy.

INVOLVEMENT IN ACADEMIC PSYCHIATRY BY PARENT ADVOCACY GROUPS

I ran into this buzzsaw myself at an annual APA meeting. My
writings usually concern the effects of ongoing dysfunctional family
interactions on the course in adults of a personality disorder called
borderline personality disorder (BPD). Studies have shown that a lot
of the more dramatic symptoms of this disorder tend to "burn out"
or ease when patients reach their forties. At my presentation at the
meeting, I made an off-the-cuff and admittedly insensitive remark to
the effect that I thought this happened because their parents were
either dying off or getting mellower as they aged. At that time, I had no
idea that family advocacy groups for parents of progeny with the disorder even came to academic presentations. I found out the hard way.

Later that evening, I attended a dinner for members of the Association for Research in Personality Disorders. During the informal
portion of the meeting prior to the dinner, a member of an organization called the National Education Alliance for Borderline Personality Disorder (NEA-BPD), one of two organizations advocating for
the families of patients with BPD, came up to me and said sharply,
"My daughter has borderline personality disorder. She's much better,
and I'm not dead!"

I spent the dinner sitting right next to her, discussing the situation and making friends with her. I apologized for the insensitive
remark, reminding her that I also had said that the parents may be
mellowing out. I tried to explain that I actually have great empathy
for the parents of individuals with BPD, even the abusive ones. I
know what they are up against, because my patients have done to
me what they do to their parents. Patients with BPD have the reputation among therapists for being the most aggravating and infuriat-
ing patients on the face of the planet, and do they ever deserve it.
Many therapists and psychiatrists hate treating them for that reason.

I believe that all members of a family share in dysfunctional
interactions. As my colleague Sylvia Landau says, they are all beans

in the same soup. At the dinner, I went on to say that my BPD patients often get angry with me because they think I am *defending* their parents. As I will describe later, I try to find something redeeming about all parents, some of whom quite frankly have done some hair-raising and horrific things to their children. Every time I think that I have heard it all, I hear something shocking and new even for me.

However, blaming even those parents who were clearly and severely abusive for the way their children turned out as adults is very counterproductive. It tends to lead the parents to act out even more of the problematic behavior in question rather than less of it, which may in turn exacerbate the problematic behavior of their grown progeny. The reason for this will be discussed later in this chapter. In the next section, I will discuss two other cultural developments that concern the issue of victimhood and blame.

THE ISSUE OF BLAME IN SPOUSE ABUSE

Another form of political correctness also reared its head around the same time as the developments discussed in the last section and also contributed to family systems theories and therapy falling out of fashion. This one has to do with spouse abuse. It was sort of the inverse of, and really incompatible with, the criticism of NAMI of "parent bashing," or blaming parents for the problems of their children. Instead of bashing the parents, advocates for the abused worry about "blaming the victim."

For decades attorneys who defended accused rapists, in order to get their accused clients acquitted, attacked female victims for having "entrapped" their hapless clients. Rape victims were said to have worn skimpy clothes that created irresistible sexual urges in men, or accused of being tramps who were known by their assailants as loose women who freely slept around. The lawyers argued that seeming victims of rape were "asking for it." The entire past sex life of the victim became fair game for cross-examination.

Following the women's liberation movement of the 1960s, when women first entered the work force in large numbers and became more powerful and influential as a group, such practices led once again to justifiable outrage in a significant portion of the population. The rape victim's past sexual practices and her taste in apparel are obviously completely invalid excuses for an inexcusable crime, and these character attacks on women have since been disallowed as evidence in court. I for one could not be happier about this now being the case.

A similar change in philosophy occurred after the extent of wife abuse in this country became widely publicized. Before then, wife beaters were often acquitted of spousal battery, if they were even prosecuted at all, by claiming that they were so provoked by the woman they had beaten that their rage had become uncontrollable and uncontainable. They said the women were to blame for their own beating. The police and the courts would often give the accused husband a wink and a nod. Abusive husbands could also avoid even the potential of charges entirely by intimidating their wives from filing a complaint. Only recently have police departments taken spousal abuse more seriously, taken photos of the bruises on the women, and prosecuted the men even if the wives refused to file a complaint or testify.

Again, I am as outraged about what used to happen as anyone, and I am not complaining at all about the changes in the public's attitude. I do not care how much someone has been provoked; this does not give him license to beat someone up. If I were a courtroom judge in such a case, the man would go to prison and the woman would walk. That is cut and dried.

The problem for family therapy came about because, due to justifiable anger over the way women have been devalued in the past, even looking at the behavior of a woman in an abusive relationship became politically incorrect. If I am a therapist who wants to help the couple change their behavior—and it is just not true that no spouse abusers ever stop, although many do continue or escalate their abuse—then the matter is not so cut and dried. Just as the systems therapists maintain, I must look at the behavior of everyone in the family.

Discussing the woman's behavior in the context of the abuse does not mean that it is her "fault" that she was abused, nor that she is a masochist who enjoys pain. However, absolving an abused woman living in the U.S. in the twenty-first century of all responsibility for her fate is counterproductive as well as spurious. This can best be illustrated by the example of a patient I once treated. She was married to an extremely hotheaded and jealous man who had beaten her severely on a few past occasions. One day in a fit of pique, she torched his prized vehicle and then had sex with his best friend. She then went home to tell him all about what she had done in the nastiest way she could think of and blamed her misbehavior on his inadequacy as a husband. Can the reader guess what happened next?

What happened next, of course, was that right after my patient's confession her husband beat her up. Let's see a show of hands: Did anyone reading this guess what was going to happen correctly? Did anyone see that coming? Does anyone really doubt that my patient knew beforehand that this would happen? She was not a stupid woman. However, *if* her goal was to avoid being beaten, her behavior was stupid. Again, this does not mean she enjoyed being beaten, so we need to come up with some other explanation.

The bizarreness of such situations is further compounded by something else abused wives frequently say. When asked by a therapist why they have not left an abusive husband, the dumbfounding reply is often "Because I love him." What? He has beaten you several times to the point where the bruises made your body look like a checkerboard, and you *love* him? That sounds crazy! Women nowadays say this less frequently than in the past because they now know that many therapists will jump on their case for making such a statement, yet they still think and feel that way.

If a therapist has heard an abused woman say this, then I think it is quite likely that her tormenter has also heard it. He, not being completely stupid, would have to ask himself, "How come you love me when I beat you up? Come to think of it, sometimes you do things that you *know* will lead to a beating. Why on earth would you do that?"

When a therapist attempts to treat an abusive husband, perhaps by court order, and asks him what makes him do what he does, he may not answer truthfully. If he were to say, "I know this sounds crazy, doc, but I think she *wants* me to beat her up. I think she loves me *because* I beat her up," he knows exactly what he would hear in response from almost any therapist. The therapist would almost certainly exhibit an angry and disgusted facial expression and accuse him, perhaps in a sugar-coated but still easy to spot way, of trying to justify his vile behavior through rationalizations and deflecting the blame for his own shortcomings onto his victim. The average abuser generally knows better than to subject himself to that unless he actively wants the therapist to hate him.

Occasionally this kind of statement comes out of the mouth of an abusive spouse anyway. One patient I observed in a videotaped therapy session, while describing what he said during an unusual violent episode with his wife, quoted himself as saying to her right before he struck her, "Is *this* what you want?"

The typical explanation for why the men who control and dominate their wives through abuse do so is that they grew up in a household where acting in this manner was expected from men. Their subculture supposedly showed them that this was the best way to maintain dominance over females, and that exhibiting such dominance was a sign that they were "real men." Often, their fathers physically abused their mothers and they witnessed that.

Therefore, these men simply did not have role models for better ways to treat women, and so they do not think there is anything wrong with beating them.

I always had trouble with this explanation. First, when I was growing up, I often heard it said by a lot of different people in many different contexts that beating a woman was the most cowardly thing a man could do. Second, when I picture a young boy watching his father beat his mother, I do not picture the boy smiling, cheering and shouting, "Way to go, Dad! The bitch deserves it!" I picture him cowering in fear and horror. How could he *not* know his father's behavior is wrong?

In many cases, I have heard male abusers speak of getting in between their father and their mother to try to stop a beating, even when they were not yet big enough to do so. As a result, they were often then badly beaten themselves. Yet somehow they grew up and beat their own wives. Why? Should not they, of all people, be the ones who really should know better? Human behavior is so damn strange.

The issue of victimhood has led to yet another cultural reaction that has affected the mental health profession in the same direction as these others. I now refer to popular revulsion with what is termed the culture of victimhood.

THE CULTURE OF VICTIMHOOD

Many people have grown tired of hearing what they perceive to be disingenuous and lame excuses for bad behavior or for major personal failings. In the popular perception, those caught red-handed committing crimes, behaving in ways that are widely disapproved, or performing their jobs carelessly with disastrous consequences want to blame everyone but themselves for what happened. They are said to refuse to take "personal responsibility" for their actions.

They blame their behavior on unhappy childhoods or bad experiences earlier in their lives. They label their obviously willful misconduct as an innocent "mistake" or an understandable "error in judgment." People who sympathize with them are called "bleeding heart liberals" and are accused of foolishly buying into their tawdry excuses. In other venues, members of some minority groups are criticized, even by black commentators like Bill Cosby, for excusing the failure of high numbers of students in inner-city schools by blaming society's racism, rather than by discussing the students' failure to study or the lack of encouragement they receive at home from their families. Lawsuits are filed claiming damages by people who have tripped over a barely hidden sprinkler head when their own carelessness, as well as the fact they were trespassing, was a major contributing factor to the accident.

On another level, the culture at large has also tired of people who, while acknowledged as having been victims of this or that, continually whine about what happened to them. Such people are accused of dwelling on the past, not moving on with their lives, and wallowing in their victimhood. Some of them do seem to wear past injustices as a badge of honor, and base their entire lives around them. "So what if they were abused as children?" cultural voices ask. "Bad things happen to everyone! They should just get over it." This type of sentiment was epitomized in the lyrics from a song by the Eagles, appropriately titled *Get Over It*. An example:

I'd like to find your inner child and kick its little ass.

Therapists would joke that they should start doing "single session therapy" by slapping their clients in the face and screaming, "Snap out of it!" like in the scene from the movie *Moonstruck*.

Believe me, most of my unhappy patients would give anything to "get over it." I want them to as well. That is the goal of their treatment. However, biological and genetic factors make getting over it very difficult, as I shall elucidate in Chapter Four. The question is not whether they should get over it, but how.

Paradoxically, some of the same individuals who believe that it is illegitimate for an individual to blame a horrific hard luck past history or a bad childhood for personal problems also themselves whine about how cultural influences have caused people to go astray. In this view, for example, pornography and violence in the media are the major causes of unsafe sex and antisocial behavior. Personal responsibility somehow does not seem to enter into this viewpoint when these issues are brought up. For example, studies are quoted that "prove" that exposure to violence on television leads to aggressive behavior and crime.

Of course, what the vast majority of these studies really show is an increase in aggressive thoughts and minor aggressive behavior immediately following viewing of film violence in some children. They do not show an increase in antisocial acts over time. As many commentators have pointed out, TV and movie violence has grown progressively and steadily more pervasive and more graphic over the last few decades, while the violent crime rate has dropped significantly at times during this same period. An argument could be made that teenagers who are watching the most TV, including violent shows, are couch potatoes, and are not the ones who are going out and getting into trouble. One very study from the early 1960s showed that children who were exposed to the shows like *The Ed Sullivan Show* committed significantly more antisocial acts that those exposed to more violent shows like *The Untouchables.*[1]

High-Profile Criminal Cases

The fires of popular disgust with the culture of victimhood were fanned when various absurd psychological excuses were seemingly used as defenses in high-profile criminal trials. The idea that a lot of criminals are literally getting away with murder due to pleading insanity is actually a myth. This form of defense tactic is seldom used and if used, seldom successful. According to CNN, Justice Department statistics show that the insanity defense is used only in approximately 1 percent of criminal cases, and less than a quarter of those eventually prove successful.

Cases in which it has been successfully used, as in John Hinckley's assassination attempt against Ronald Reagan in 1981, often receive a raft of publicity. In Hinckley's case, it led to a large public outcry, despite the fact that Hinckley was clearly psychotic. Ironically, individuals who are successful with an insanity defense are often locked in psychiatric hospitals for much longer periods than the time they would have spent in a jail sentence for their crime.

Another high-profile case was that of Dan White, who assassinated San Francisco Mayor George Moscone and Supervisor Harvey Milk in 1978. He received a light sentence after his lawyers employed a strategy that became known as the "Twinkie defense." The public perception was that his lawyers argued that he was not in his right mind and therefore had what is termed *diminished capacity* because of a high blood sugar level caused by eating too much junk food. In truth, the lawyers argued that his eating too much junk food was a symptom of depression, and that it was his depression that led to the diminished capacity, not the junk food per se. However, that is not what the public heard. Despite popular ridicule of White's defense, many parents at that time believed that too much sugar could adversely affect behavior, at least in their children.

These cases occurred quite a long time ago, but they are still frequently brought up by the media and continue to exert strong effects on public opinion. The power of high-profile news stories to shape public opinion for a long time when most people have no personal memories of the events that occurred or of subsequent events, and have not been exposed to differing accounts of what took place, should not be underestimated. When I moved to Memphis in 1992, for example, some of my baby boomer friends in my hometown of Los Angeles still pictured the South as being just like they had seen it on television decades ago at the time of the integration of Ole Miss and Little Rock's Central High School.

Another major cultural phenomenon that has diminished the influence of psychotherapies that deal with dysfunctional families is the massive increase in parental guilt over the last few decades about their relationship with their children and its effects on the way children are raised. That is the subject of the next section.

GUILTY PARENTS

The popular parenting advice columnist John Rosemond describes an epidemic of poor parenting practices that has been accompanied by an epidemic of out-of-control children. For instance, he notes that behavior such as children biting their parents has become increasingly common. As an antidote, he promotes "traditional" parenting. He pines for the day in which the parents' relationship with each other was of more overall importance to them than their relationship with their children, when parents did not try to be friends with their kids, when parents did not see their children as direct reflections of their personal adequacy, when parents did not believe that if they were sufficiently attentive to their children then the children would automatically be successful, and when parents did not try to reason or bargain with two-year-olds.

I wholeheartedly agree with Rosemond that these changes have been very destructive and have contributed to an increase in emotional and behavioral problems in children that will continue for years. I believe they are behind such phenomena as the increase in binge drinking among college students. What is behind the change in parenting practices? The explanation I propose is that a very sudden and all-encompassing cultural shift has led to a dramatic increase in the level of guilt among parents. The guilt has in turn led an increasing number of parents to be oversolicitous of and afraid to discipline their children. The kids *act out* in response, which then causes the parents to get angry with them.

Acting out is defined as performing an action to express often subconscious emotional conflicts. Acting out usually consists of out-of-control aggressive or sexual behavior that is engaged in to gain relief from tension or anxiety. Impulses to act out often result in antisocial, combative, rude, oppositional, or hyperactive behavior.

The parenting patterns I am about to describe do not necessarily correlate on a one-to-one basis with the emotional problems of parents' children. As we shall see later, no single causative factor is either necessary or sufficient to produce the vast majority of psychiatric conditions and behavior problems. Dysfunctional patterns themselves vary widely in severity and pervasiveness, and they are counterbalanced by a multitude of other biological, psychological, and social factors, which themselves vary widely on those same dimensions. Nonetheless, some common themes have emerged.

A Massive Cultural Change

The women's movement, combined with economic changes that made surviving on only one income increasingly difficult for families, led to one of the fastest and most massive cultural shifts in history. Almost overnight, women entered the work force in huge numbers. Female ambition was fully unleashed for the first time ever, and flourished. However, women who wanted to get to the top in their field in business and the professions ran into a roadblock. They found that, in the business and professional worlds, they had to act just like the men in one respect. They could not use the needs of their children as a reason for refusing to put in the long hours necessary in today's economy to climb the corporate ladder. The United States had during this same period of time grown to become the most workaholic country on Earth, eventually surpassing even Japan.

Women who wanted to and who were told that they could "have it all" by the ambient culture found that doing so was not as easy as some famous women made it look. Since their husbands were only just beginning to share in child care and were as much or more involved with their careers as they ever had been, who would be around to take care of the children? Horror stories about bad things happening to "latchkey children," left to their own devices and locked in their homes without parental supervision after school, began to circulate.

Debate over working mothers became one of the most important theaters of operations in the culture wars that continue to rage to this day. Reactionary forces that never believed in equality for women in the first place began to spout off about all the damage being done by working mothers to their offspring. The voices of people like Phyllis Schlafly, a career woman who made a career out of attacking career women, became louder and more shrill. Unfortunately, researchers in major academic centers began to give voices like hers more ammunition.

Widely publicized studies showed that, on average, children in families in which at least one parent stayed home with them did better in life on some dimensions than those children from families in which this was not the case. Of course, many children of two-career families do splendidly or even better than many of their more closely parented peers, while many children of stay-at-home mothers often fail spectacularly in life, but the press ignored the scatter and put most of its focus on the "average" end result.

The various reactions to the rapid shift in cultural demands and the resultant media reports mentioned above—taking place before the logistics of "having it all" could be worked out and families had much time to adjust their value systems—resulted in a wide variety of new family behavior patterns. Of course, many families were able to negotiate the cultural changes successfully and continued to calmly set limits with their children while encouraging them to have egalitarian attitudes toward gender roles. The family behavior patterns and individual reactions that I am about to describe constitute those that are perhaps the most common ones that I have encountered in my patients with personality and relationship difficulties, but they are hardly the only ones.

Many working mothers were already experiencing a vague sense of guilt about their absences from the home even before the media backlash. The media currents and the increasing time demands from employers made this preexisting guilt even worse. The original source of the ill-defined guilt was far more insidious and devastating than the other factors.

Many career women found that they were faced with considerable criticism about their choices in life from within their own families. The baby boomers, who were the first large wave of career women, had themselves been raised by parents from the World War II "greatest" generation. This earlier generation of women had been, on the whole, raised to conform to the old female gender role stereotypes. They were taught that they were supposed to be totally fulfilled by being nothing but wives and mothers, as their mothers had been before them. However, unlike their own mothers, some of these women had had a taste of career fulfillment during the war.

When all of the men were shipped off to Europe and the Pacific, few were left at home to help build the needed machines of war. The "Rosie the Riveter" phenomenon was born. Women took the jobs the men had left behind, and many found the experience exhilarating. As soon as the war was over and the men returned, however, they were told to go home and to be nothing more than wives and mothers once again. The U.S. government actually made propaganda films whose basic message was, for all intents and purposes, "Great job, girls, but it's time to go back home and get barefoot and pregnant once again." By today's standards, these films were horrifically sexist and are positively dumbfounding to watch. Few apparently thought so at the time. Women followed the instructions in the films, and the baby boom ensued.

Since these women had been raised from birth to believe in the old roles, they accepted their fate, at least on the outside. Inside, many of them subconsciously resented having to give up the excitement of their careers. Some carried this covert resentment with them for the rest of their lives. As parents are wont to do, they tried to vicariously experience what they were missing through their children. When they had daughters, they often pushed the girls to go out and get what had been denied to them: a satisfying career. Perhaps it was no accident that the baby boom generation was at the forefront of the feminist movement of the 1960s. Feminism had been an undercurrent in society for decades before then, but "women's lib" virtually exploded.

As the female boomers hobnobbed with one another and talked among themselves about how women could now do anything they wanted, many faced a rather disturbing negative reaction from both of their parents when they spoke about this at home. The parents would suddenly become hostile and/or withdrawn, sometimes for no apparent reason.

Many male boomers, on the other hand, were the objects of some strange reactions from their parents as well. They had started to realize that sharing the burdens of being the family breadwinner was not such a bad idea after all. However, their fathers seemed to think less of them if they were not dominant over their wives. Some of their mothers acted helpless and dependent around them at times, but because of the mothers' covert resentment at males for keeping them from careers, they emasculated the sons who tried to take care of them in any way. For example, one of my patients told of an incident in which his World War II generation grandmother fell in the bathroom and broke her hip. When my patient tried to come to her aid, she refused to unlock the bathroom door. She said that she did not want to be a bother.

These parents were not being mean-spirited when they acted like this. The parents had grown up with certain gender role expectations and believed in them. They also worried, because of their own experiences, that successful women might have a difficult time finding a mate. They believed that men would find feminists too aggressive, and in any event would be threatened by a female who might make more money than they did. These fears were stoked to near hysteria among both the boomers and their parents by a story in *Newsweek* in 1986, since discredited, that purported to show that college-educated women who were still single at the age of thirty-five had only a 5 percent chance of ever getting married.

More important than the possible reactions of male chauvinist peers, the parents of the boomers, just like their children, worried about what might happen to their grandchildren if one of their parents were not in the home to raise them as much as in past generations. How would such children fare in life?

In addition to this concern, a covert but pernicious issue lurked in the back of the minds of a significant number of the former riveting Rosies. When their daughters became successful in business, the mothers were reminded of what they themselves had given up right after the war. They had pretended for many years that having given up their jobs was really no big deal to them. They did this so as not to upset their husbands and their own parents. For them to switch gears and to suddenly become supportive of their daughters' career ambitions now might expose their deceit. Nonetheless they felt envious of their daughters. In response, some just became quiet, some became depressed, and others became actively critical of their daughters' ambitions, especially when grandchildren came into the picture.

Boomer females were extremely confused by their parents' mixed message, which seemed to say, "I'm so proud of you for your career success, but stop doing what you're doing." Many were left with a highly unsettling feeling caused by this strange lack of support. They wanted and planned to go on with their careers, but somehow they did not feel quite right about it. They became somewhat confused about exactly what their role in life should look like. Men found that they were criticized by their girlfriends if they opened a car door for a woman or if they did not. Accompanying the role confusion for both sexes was the nagging, unnamed sense of guilt about their children that was mentioned above, which was then further increased by the other cultural developments.

Paradoxically, the existence of parental guilt of this magnitude had effects on parenting behavior that may be the real reason why children of two-career families do slightly worse than those with stay-at-home mothers. These changes in parenting style driven by guilt are probably far more destructive to children than the fact that both parents are working per se.

The guilt and the role confusion in turn affected the next generation. Both girls and boys in that next group saw that dual-career families were becoming the norm, but they also had not been completely supported for proceeding with it themselves by their unsure and insecure parents. They were excited by the possibility of having it all, but afraid of the prospect at the same time. The evolution of gender role confusion is a good example of the process through which anxiety and ambivalence about cultural changes are passed down from one generation to the next, while the original source of the anxiety is hidden from the younger generation.

All of this confusion and ambivalence created two different groups of women who, while superficially polar opposites from one another, shared the exact same conflict. One group had careers but covertly envied the stay-at-home mothers, while a second group stayed at home with their children but covertly envied the career women. The latter group also had quite secret—or so they thought—deep-seated urges to escape the drudgery of doing housework and shuttling children around all day long.

Guilty Behavior

Many parents in two-career families worried covertly but obsessively that they were short-changing their own children. Some stay-at-home mothers, on the other hand, subconsciously worried that their hidden resentment over their burdens and their choices in life might adversely affect their children. In response, both of these groups began to monitor their children carefully for any sign of distress that might indicate even the slightest parental failing. A good percentage of them became so obsessed with their children that they spent every spare moment with them, sometimes at the expense of their marriage.

Both groups subtly disparaged those couples who solved this dilemma by simply refusing to have any children. Such couples were referred to disapprovingly as DINKS (double income, no kids) and were accusing of being "selfish." Still, the conflicted parents' envy of the DINKS was palpable.

For the career women, the guiltier they felt, the more concerned they became with turning any time they did spend with their children into "quality time." They tried to make up for their frequent absences to their children by catering to their every whim. The stay-at-home mothers began to do the exact same thing. They also became overcome with guilt as their resentment over the perceived drudgery of their life, as well as their hidden desires to escape from it, built up over time.

Their poor dears were not allowed to be even slightly uncomfortable for even a minute. If they cried, the parents' job number one was to make sure that they felt better immediately. Very few demands were made on children for chores. If children disobeyed, they were punished inconsistently if at all. The parents secretly feared that punishing the children's misbehavior might be doing even more damage to their children than that already being caused by either their frequent unavailability or their hidden anger. Instead, they tried to give rewards for "good" behavior in the form of increasingly elaborate material goodies, but never knew when to stop. The children's rooms began to look like "Toys 'R You Guys."

In many of these families, couples began to literally compete with one another about which of them had raised the most gifted, talented, successful, and well-rounded children, in order to prove to everyone, including themselves, that they were good parents in spite of their careers or their repressed ambition. The more affluent ones began to run their children ragged with almost daily lessons in music and various athletic endeavors such as ice skating or gymnastics, spending enormous sums of money in the process. Throwing lavish birthday parties in which no expense was spared became a competitive sport. The free playtime so ubiquitous in the fifties and early sixties, when neighborhood kids on roller skates and bikes enjoyed each others' company all afternoon, began to disappear from the cultural landscape.

A cottage industry of "prestige" preschools and private grade schools arose to take advantage of increasingly desperate parents. Screening interviews and rejection slips for toddlers, modeled after those from Ivy League colleges, were designed to artificially inflate demand. Parents whose kids did not make the cut would begin to worry about whether or not they had been adequate parents.

Conflicted stay-at-home mothers, in order to prove to themselves that they had made the right choice, threw themselves into serving their children. For instance, they might decide to homeschool them. Additionally, instead of allowing them to freely play outside with other children, they would organize "playdates" with the children of like-minded moms and dads. The parents would always be present in the next room to keep an eye on things. They would rationalize that spending so much time with their children would prevent the little ones from being exposed to corrupting cultural influences, perhaps all of that left-wing godless women's lib stuff. Unfortunately, as they did more and more for their children and less and less for themselves, they began to resent their children even more.

Everything that happened in the home began to center around the children. John Rosemond's nightmare world of nontraditional parenting was born.

Cultural Lag

The effect on individual families of the historical process in which the roles of women and parents changed drastically over a short period of time is a good example of what anthropologists term *cultural lag*. Cultural lag means that the rules by which families operate, and the definitions of the roles that each family member plays within the family, do not keep up with changes demanded by changes in the larger culture. Such cultural events as the sudden need for families to have two wage earners to survive necessitate different sorts of family rules and roles than those that were previously acceptable.

Cultural lag creates a situation where members of some families, particularly the younger ones, are exposed to enticing ideas that are threatening to older family members. In this case, the roles of women were changing so fast that large numbers of families were left in the dust. People became torn between their personal desires to partake in the opportunities created by the new culture and their loyalty to their family. These opposing forces led to severe *ambivalence* in individuals about how they should behave in certain contexts. Psychoanalysts refer to severe ambivalence as *intrapsychic conflict*, although they do not necessarily conceptualize it in quite the way I am describing.

For reasons to be discussed in a later chapter, children raised in a family environment ridden with parental guilt begin to act out. When children start to act out, the parents' guilt causes them to blame themselves for the children's problems and misbehavior. In response, the parents pull back even more from effective discipline and limit setting, which in turn further increases acting out by the children.

Observing their out-of-control grandchildren also gave the career parents' own parents reason to believe that their offspring's career emphasis was having deleterious effects on their families. This concern often led them to further increase their verbal criticisms of their children's parenting priorities, which then created yet more guilt in the parents. Simultaneously with all these events, career demands continued to pile up; working parents began to feel crushed by their dilemma and their responsibilities.

Conversely, the mothers of stay-at-home parents who had repressed ambitions of their own, and who were deprived of the opportunity to live vicariously through their daughters, started to level thinly veiled criticisms of their daughters' decision to not have a career. Anxiety created by this mixed message would then further feed into their daughters' resentment of their children, which in turn also fueled more guilt.

Divorce

In those situations where parents divorced, parental guilt was again severely aggravated. Studies and newspaper stories began to come out showing that children of divorced and blended families did, on average, somewhat worse than those from intact families. Hearing about this, the grandparents, who came from a generation in which divorce was less common than it is today, might add guilt trips about divorce to their already impressive list of guilt-inducing behaviors. The mother of one patient of mine, who finally decided to get out of a long-term loveless marriage, shouted at her, "You are going to destroy your children!"

Divorced parents thusly affected began to ruminate about the possibility that their divorce was causing irreparable harm to their kids. They would covertly feel even more responsible for and even more guilty about any problems their children might have. Parents began to oscillate between taking over yet more aspects of their children's lives and trying to foist their children off on someone else in order to escape from all of their noxious feelings.

When they remarried, these mixed feelings could lead to significant marital problems with a new spouse. They would initially ask their new spouse to help with the disciplining of his or her stepchildren. However, because of the guilt, the biological parents would often interfere with this process and without warning step in to take over the discipline themselves, while criticizing the stepparent for not doing it right. This put stepparents in a no-win situation. They would be criticized regardless of whether they pitched in with disciplining the stepchildren or if they refrained from doing so. The couple would have difficulty coming to any agreement about how to handle the children. In turn, the increased tension in the new marriage would upset the children and lead to yet more acting out.

In earlier generations, custody of children from divorcing families in the United States was routinely granted to the mother. In order to lose custody, the mother would practically have to abandon the child or go out and become a prostitute. With the rise of feminism, paradoxically, this attitude of the courts changed. Fathers began demanding and being awarded custody. Worried that their divorce would damage their children and not wanting to feel personally responsible, each member of the divorcing couples would blame the other for the marital split and for any behavior problems their children had that might have resulted from it. Divorces and custody battles became on average nastier and nastier, with each parent often trying to poison the mind of the child against the other parent. The involved children would be torn apart by divided loyalties. In response, new behavioral problems would surface, and any preexisting behavior problem they had would worsen.

Mounting Frustration

Frustration with their children, work stress, and family criticism mounted to unbearable levels, and some affected parents eventually lost control and at times went into a blind rage. Child abuse was sometimes the result. Other parents went to the opposite extreme and metaphorically ran for the hills, leading their children to be neglected. Still others went back and forth between hostile overinvolvement and hostile underinvolvement. Many began to look for a scapegoat for their children's misbehavior, so they would not have to feel all of that horrible guilt.

If a child became hyperactive and disrespectful, perhaps the fault lay not in their own absences from the home and their other obligations, but because the child had a defective brain. They became entranced by the pied pipers of biological child psychiatry who offered explanations for their children's behavior that did not include problematic parenting practices. They tried to convince themselves, often rather unsuccessfully, that they were not in any way at fault. Other parents who disapproved of psychiatry or psychiatric medication might instead blame the problems of their children on food additives or sugar. Despite studies that almost unanimously disprove those theories, many parents still believe in them.

If their children had academic or discipline problems in school, some parents blamed the teachers for having unreasonable expectations or for being just plain mean. Teachers were at times accused of lying about the children's behavior. In the not-too-distant past, when a teacher sent a note home describing a child's misbehavior in school, parents would punish the child even more than the school did. Now, they may instead attack the teacher. School administrators often want to get the complaining parents off of their backs and offer little support to the innocent teachers.

The guilty concerns of parents over their adequacy as parents did not stop when their children became older, but continued to affect parental behavior as the children became adolescents and grownups. In some of the more severely affected families, parents would repeatedly bail out acting-out children from one self-inflicted crisis after another. For example, they might pay thousands of dollars for multiple drug rehabilitation programs for their progeny despite the fact that their child repeatedly signed out of the programs prematurely with some ridiculous excuse and then continued to use drugs. They believed their children's explanation that they had left treatment because they were being unfairly treated, and blamed the program's "failure" on the policies of the facility.

Alternatively, parents would allow their teens to be placed in psychiatric hospitals, where shrewd but unethical hospital administrators and psychiatrists blamed the adolescent's emotional problems and misbehavior, or even their suicide attempts, on cultural phenomena such as heavy metal music. This way, the parents would not feel that they were being scrutinized or blamed, and would gladly pay up. Some hospitalized kids were kept there for months until their insurance ran out and then summarily discharged. *Peer pressure* was another scapegoat offered up by hospitals to these parents. Of course peers do have a significant influence on teenagers, but with which peers adolescents choose to associate is no accident of fate.

When their teenagers get older, some guilty parents become what college administrators and employers refer to as "helicopter parents." Such parents literally hover over their adult offspring trying to keep their lives on track, and personally deal with anyone in a position of authority over them in order to make certain their little darlings are treated right. This of course leads their children to avoid learning to become responsible for themselves.

One other interesting phenomenon I witnessed when I was practicing in Los Angeles in the 1980s may also be related to widespread parental guilt. I have not seen it since I moved to Memphis, although it still may be taking place. Some parents became what I referred to as the "neighborhood den mothers for dysfunctional children." The home of a parent whose teenage child had had emotional problems, dropped out of school, or had gotten into drugs became the gathering place for several other teens with similar problems.

The den mothers, most of whom had been stay-at-home moms for their kids, would lend a sympathetic ear to all of the "adoptees," especially when the teens complained about their frequently absent parents. Perhaps the den mothers felt compelled to prove they were great parents by compulsively catering to all the other kids who were having similar problems to the ones their kids had, and then blaming the problems on the working mothers.

THE COUNTERPRODUCTIVENESS OF BLAMING PARENTS

If many problematic parenting practices are indeed based on guilt, one can easily see why blaming parents for the way their children have turned out makes family problems worse rather than better. It adds to the already unmanageable guilt these parents are struggling with, and makes them try even harder to prove to the world that they had been good parents by further "protecting" their kids from adversity. This hyperconcern is what fuels many of the problem interactions they have with their children in the first place, and feeling blamed makes them stick to them even more tightly. This paradox sets up a bind for family therapists: How do we help parents look at and be responsible for their own actions without making them feel guiltier than they already do? Achieving this goal requires a real tightrope walk by a therapist.

John Rosemond does a brilliant job of avoiding the guilt issue in his advice column, even while complaining bitterly about today's parenting practices. He tells parents that their children have minds of their own, and that parents are but one of many influences that affect how children turn out. He often goes on to say that even the children of the best parents in the world can turn into adults who have all kinds of behavioral problems, and that children can still turn out well in spite of severe family discord or even abuse.

This is all true to a point. However, Rosemond then proceeds to offer parenting solutions that, if enacted, will probably solve the behavioral problem about which the parents are complaining, although he offers no guarantee. Of course, if the problem can be changed by changing parental behavior, this implies that their behavior might be at least partially responsible for it in the first place.

A good example of his technique appeared in Rosemond's newspaper column on September 18, 2008. A divorced mother wrote in asking for advice about how she should talk to her thirteen-year-old daughter when the daughter complained about her father's irresponsibility about keeping promises to the girl. The mother had gone out of her way to tell her daughter several times not to speak ill of him. Rosemond correctly ascertained that the mother's excessive focus on the topic was inadvertently feeding into the daughter's resentment of her father, and furthermore that the daughter knew very well that the mother gave the advice she did only because she felt it was the right thing to say, not because the mother really was not herself angry at the father's behavior. I would also wonder if beneath Mom's almost obsessive concern with the issue lurked her own guilt over the fact that she had married the bum, or over any ill effects the parental divorce may have had on her daughter.

After assuring the mother that parenting was only one influence among many on the girl, Rosemond suggested that the mother help the girl get "unstuck" by telling her that everything about the father's irresponsibility had already been discussed, and that therefore they would have no more conversations about it. The daughter was just going to have to deal with the situation on her own from that point on.

This strategy is similar to the strategy used by Al-Anon to get relatives of alcoholics to quit enabling them. Their motto is "Let go and let God." By this they mean that relatives should stop trying to "fix" the alcoholic and leave that chore in God's hands. If the relatives buy into this, they stop their enabling behavior. Doing so actually may help the alcoholic to change his drinking habits. In other words, by changing their own behavior through *not* trying to stop an alcoholic from destroying himself, they are behaving in ways which may very well help the alcoholic, while simultaneously feeling entirely blameless for having formerly enabled him. Their letting go and letting God, if enacted, does not always work, of course, but it stands a better chance than anything else of helping their alcoholic relative to stop drinking.

Most guilty parents have not been lucky enough to get the right sort of help. They become hypersensitive about their parenting practices and brook no criticism of their children. These couples may themselves be highly critical of anyone else who does not raise their children in the exact same way that they do. The surest way to start a war in a public place is for someone to come up to a mother and tell her she is not doing right by her child. Restaurant patrons who complain to the parents at the next table about kids running amok and disturbing the other diners take their lives in their hands.

Despite the fact that such hypersensitive parents are, at least in private, highly critical of the parenting of other people, they paradoxically become very nervous when anyone suggests that the wrong type of parenting might, in general, have an adverse effect on children. They panic at the thought that maybe what they are doing with their children might not be right after all. This pattern of defensiveness was at least in part responsible for the development of a subculture that denigrated and invalidated adults who claimed that they had emotional problems because their parents had been abusive to them when they were children. This is the subject of the next chapter.

3

The "Abuse Excuse" Revisited

Starting in the mid-1990s, a tremendous backlash developed against the previous decade's revelations about the extent of child abuse in the United States. This backlash extended to scientists who showed that child abuse was highly prevalent in the backgrounds of individuals suffering from a variety of psychiatric disorders such as eating disorders, anxiety disorders, post-traumatic stress disorders, affective disorders, and personality disorders.

Perhaps because American parents were frightened of seeing themselves in a negative light for all the reasons discussed in the previous chapter, the popular press as well as parent advocacy groups began to look for alternate explanations for the rash of abuse accusations. A commonly heard argument was that people were making up the stories about abuse because they were trying to deflect criticism of their own inadequacies, or because they had become victims of unscrupulous therapists who planted false memories in them.

CONTROVERSIES ABOUT THE PREVALENCE OF CHILD ABUSE

That child abuse takes place and is fairly common in the United States is an established fact, despite protestations to the contrary. We can look at verifiable statistics. According to *Child Maltreatment 2006*, a recent report of data from the National Child Abuse and Neglect Data System (NCANDS), approximately 905,000 children were found with reasonable legal certainty to be victims of child abuse or neglect in federal fiscal year 2006. This represents a rate of 12.1 per 1,000 children in the population. In 2003, there were 906,000 child abuse convictions. On average, there are over 3 million reports of child abuse made annually. For 2006, the rate was 47.8 reports per 1,000 children: an estimated 3,573,000 children. This means that close to one-third of reports lead to an actual conviction. Many of the other cases may still have been valid, but not enough evidence could be uncovered by the authorities.

The NCANDS also reported an estimated 1,530 child fatalities at the hands of caretakers in 2006. This translates to a rate of 2.04 children per 100,000 children in the general population. NCANDS defines "child fatality" as the death of a child caused by an injury resulting from abuse or neglect, or where abuse or neglect was a contributing factor. Obviously, only a very tiny percentage of child abuse or neglect ends in the death of the child.

An abuse rate of a little over 1 percent per year may seem to mean that a very small percentage of individuals have been the victims of childhood abuse, even though in aggregate the numbers are staggering. Reported child sexual abuse rates are even smaller; only 8.8 percent of the abuse convictions involved sexual abuse. Again, however, the vast majority of abuse cases are not reported because they are understandably kept hidden by the families in which they take place. Therefore, all of these data most likely represent the tip of the iceberg.

Although no one can be certain, the rate of child abuse in the United States has been estimated by some agencies to be three times greater than reported. Even cases that come to the attention of someone outside of the family often go unreported. That such is the case was illustrated by a recent survey of pediatricians, in which 27 percent said they were unlikely to report abuse as required by law even if they thought the abuse was "likely" or "very likely."[1] The percentage of abuse histories in patients who seek treatment for psychiatric disorders is a great deal higher than in the general population, because a history of child abuse is a major risk factor for the development of a variety of psychiatric problems in adulthood.

Why then would so many people express such disbelief in the veracity of abuse claims, and imply that people who accused their parents of abuse were victims of faulty or implanted memories? How about the children that were killed by their parents? Did these children just imagine or make up the fact that they were dead?

Exaggeration of the Extent of the Problem

Abused individuals as well as their advocates bear some responsibility for harming their own cause. The extent of the abuse problem, instead of being minimized as it had been before the rash of abuse statistics became widely known, has at times been wildly exaggerated. One estimate[2] asserted that the combined incidence of verbal, psychological, physical, and sexual abuse in the childhoods of individuals in this country is 80 percent!

Child abuse was "defined downwards" to include the most insignificant of infractions, something that we still see today. The *Dr. Phil* television show on September 18, 2008, featured the case of a mother who was accused by authorities of child endangerment because she had left her two-year-old child in a car for a couple of minutes to go 30 feet away to deposit some money in a Salvation Army can. She had never lost sight of the child, and it was sleeting outside, yet she was actually arrested.

It seemed that many people could not differentiate between a light spanking and a vicious beating. Some sexual abuse statistics counted cases of parents stroking a child's leg. If someone even appeared to be trying to make sexual contact but did not, that has also been counted in some estimates. A case of a father accidently brushing against his teenage daughter's breasts might be counted as a case of sexual abuse if any doubt at all existed about whether or not the contact was accidental. Fathers became afraid to hug their own daughters for fear of being accused of incest.

Why did those who actually were abused and their advocates exaggerate in such a manner? My guess is that victims (or "survivors") of significant abuse secretly want to think that their families are not as sick or evil as the abuse might suggest, and therefore want to believe that almost any parent acts that way at one time or another. In a sense, they may have been trying to normalize and depathologize their parents' abusive behavior for this reason, and in the process make their parents seem more human to them.

We also know that a significant percentage of abuse victims go on to abuse their own children. Some theorists opine that such individuals exaggerate the prevalence of child abuse because they are trying to normalize and depathologize their own behavior so they do not have to feel bad about it.

An alternate view is that they are trying to protect their parents from their own anger. They in a sense are saying to themselves, "If I'm just like them, who am I to criticize them?" The idea that victims of parental abuse may want to protect their families—an altruistic rather than a selfish motive for their behavior—may seem at first to be far-fetched. I urge the reader to keep an open mind about the idea that a form of altruism may be a very common motive for dysfunctional and destructive behavior, as this idea will be discussed extensively in this volume.

As for the advocates for the abused, they have a financial incentive to exaggerate the problem. If the problem is perceived as being very large, funding for research and "treatment" becomes more readily available. Therapists can build their practices more easily if they became abuse "specialists" due to an influx of new patients who believe that they have been abused.

Overzealous Therapists

The extreme claims of the incidence and prevalence of child abuse are clearly ludicrous, which leads some individuals to think instead that *most* abuse claims are therefore suspect. On top of that, certain mental health professionals began to claim that any and all individuals who suffer from one or another mental disorder such as bulimia (an eating disorder characterized by binging on food and self-induced vomiting) *must* have been sexually abused, even if at first patients vehemently deny such a history. Studies do not support this position at all; the vast majority of patients with any of these psychiatric disorders have not been sexually abused as children. However, some therapists who treated bulimic patients and patients with other disorders began to strongly push their patients to "remember" being abused simply because they believed the abuse just had to be there. In this line of reasoning, the lack of memory simply must have been caused by "repression."

When therapists act in such a leading and suggestive manner with children, the results can prove ludicrous as well as alarming. Children have been shown in studies to be easily induced to tell adults whatever they think the adult wants to hear under such pressure. In order to please a therapist, they can even be induced to tell tall tales of extremely improbable events, often leading to witch hunts.

A prime example was the infamous McMartin Pre-School investigations in southern California starting in 1983, during which children eventually told wild stories about having taken field trips to participate in child pornographic movies and photographs, none of which was ever found. An HBO movie recounted the sensational events and strongly implied that all of the adults who were charged were completely innocent. The mother who made the initial complaint was allegedly psychotic. The social workers who interviewed the children had prodded them repeatedly to change their initial stories in which they had actually denied any abuse, and to tell the "truth."

With adults under the influence of a therapist, the situation is a bit trickier, but again, critics had an easy time making the case that therapists were taking advantage of highly suggestible patients and implanting false memories in their clients. As many readers already know, many individuals in therapy claim that they had completely "forgotten" traumatic events from childhood and then suddenly remembered them as an adult. The issue of "recovered memories" became a focus of extreme controversy and was written about, discussed, and debated ad nauseum in a variety of media and professional contexts. A risk of rehashing arguments with which the reader is already quite familiar, allow me to review some of the arguments that were made and add my own two cents.

THE RECOVERED MEMORY DEBATE

In some incidents of "recovered memories," such memories were in fact triggered when the patient was under the influence of a psychotherapist, some of whom, as was mentioned, were a bit overzealous about believing that the patients' particular psychiatric disorder "proved" that they must have been abused. Worse yet, some of these memories had emerged when the patient was under the influence of hypnosis or the drug sodium amytal. Patients under the influence of hypnosis or amytal become highly suggestible and therefore much more vulnerable to the therapist's influence. Memories that are retrieved under these circumstances are highly unreliable. A crusading therapist may therefore seem to have "implanted" traumatic memories in patients who are "under the influence."

In one case from 1994 that was famous among psychotherapists, a wine company executive named Gary Ramona successfully sued his daughter's psychotherapists because, he alleged, the therapists persuaded his daughter that he had sexually abused her as a child. He alleged that her false accusation of incest had cost him his marriage, livelihood, and reputation. According to the suit, the therapists had implanted false memories in the depressed, bulimic girl by misinforming her that eating disorders are usually caused by childhood sexual abuse and by telling her that during a sodium amytal interview. He won his case even though the girl's mother believed that her daughter's accusations were truthful.

The Freudian Unconscious

The concept of recovered memories is based on the Freudian concepts of *repression* and the *unconscious*. Under this conceptualization, traumatic painful memories, which some studies do show are handled differently by the brain than are other memories, are somehow pushed out of a patient's awareness and become "unconscious." Freudian psychoanalysts speak of "*the* unconscious" as if it were part of the brain to which such memories are relegated. No such actual brain locale exists. The unconscious is a metaphor, not a real place.

We are of course not immediately aware of many things stored in our minds, or of processes going on within our bodies. Unless we pointedly pay attention to it, we are unaware of our breathing. One is not immediately aware of facts such as one's mother's maiden name, or a million other facts or memories, unless one is thinking about them in the present. Most of us have had the experience of having driven a familiar stretch of road lost in thought, and suddenly realizing that we have no memories of the actual trip. Psychoanalytic theory posited that those memories that are easy for the individual to retrieve or recall are *preconscious*, as opposed to unconscious. Unconscious thoughts were believed to be irretrievable.

A major difficulty with the Freudian formulation is: Where exactly do we draw the line between unconscious and preconscious? How do we know if a memory is truly irretrievable, or if instead for some reason we are just unable to bring it up to awareness at a given point in time? Sometimes we have something on "the tip of our tongue" but just cannot think of it.

Complicating this matter exponentially, in many instances individuals are motivated to deceive others for ulterior purposes. If they say they cannot remember something, is this true? How would we know if they were lying? Psychoanalysts add even further to this confusion by theorizing about other mechanisms by which we defend ourselves from thinking uncomfortable thoughts: *dissociation, suppression,* and *denial.* According to analysts, we *suppress* thoughts that we are aware of but with which we are uncomfortable. *Dissociation* means sort of going off into never-never land to avoid thinking uncomfortable thoughts.

The precise difference between a repressed or suppressed thought and a dissociated thought in psychoanalysis is somewhat hard to define in words. Analysts invoke spatial metaphors. Repression is thought of as pushing thoughts "down" (vertically), while dissociation involves a "walling off" process (horizontally). Where these spatial metaphors come from is unclear, and as the late critic Jay Haley pointed out, they are nonsensical if one really thinks about them. But even assuming they are different things, how can we really be sure if a professed lack of memory is due to repression, suppression, dissociation, or downright lying? And then the concept of *denial* rears its ugly head.

The trickiest issue of all is how to understand the fact that there are indeed facts, memories, observations, and even implications of observations that we may not *want* to remember or think about for whatever reason. Are they really irretrievable? A wife may claim that she has no idea that her husband is having an affair, even while admitting having scrubbed strange lipstick off of his shirt collar as she did the laundry. Is she truly "unconscious" of the possible implications of the lipstick? Is she just lying to herself? After all, it is quite true that human beings do lie to themselves. We are the only organisms on Earth that do that.

On the other hand, perhaps she is quite conscious of the implications and not lying to herself, but lying to us. Could she perhaps be too ashamed of herself to *admit* that she *wants* to ignore the evidence, because she thinks she deserves to be mistreated? Another individual has no way of knowing for sure which of these, or many other, possibilities is correct.

The concept of denial perfectly illustrates the difficulty in knowing the truth of a described memory or a statement that an individual makes about a memory. These days, denial has almost come to mean the exact opposite of what it actually means. If you deny that you did something, you might be "in denial," which means you actually did do it. Alcoholics, in the most obvious example, are famous for stating, "I can quit drinking any time I want." They are often said to be "in denial" about their inability to stop drinking, because their behavior suggests that they are unable to stop.

An alternate explanation—one that I happen to believe—is that such a statement does not represent "denial" at all, although the alcoholic may *want others to believe* that he or she really cannot stop. I think people who make this statement are telling the truth. I believe they are able to stop any time they want, even if they are physically addicted. They just do not want to. As I pointed out in a previous work,[3] addicted and already intoxicated individuals would have no trouble putting down a glass of booze, assuming they were not overtly suicidal, if they believed that someone would shoot them if they took the drink. As this admittedly hypothetical example illustrates, they definitely have the ability to stop their drinking, even while intoxicated. So how can we be sure what is going on in the head of someone who makes a statement like "I can stop any time I want"? We cannot.

Some might protest this example by pointing out that under longer-term circumstances, addicts cannot stop because they would go through withdrawal. However, people can be medically treated for alcohol withdrawal, yet they choose not to go this route. Even if this treatment were unavailable, as it is with opiate addiction, ask yourself what you would do if someone held you down for two weeks and injected you daily with heroin, causing you to become addicted. If you were then freed, what would you rather do next: become a heroin addict, or go through three or four days of really bad flulike symptoms?

Who's Lying and Who's Telling the Truth?

Commentators who think the concept of repression and "recovered" memories is bunk often point to sensational cases in the courts or in the press that seem to prove them right. Comedienne Roseanne Barr, for example, went public with abuse accusations against her parents and claimed to have specific memories of being sexually abused by her father when she was only six months old. Since no one has or can have memories from this age, critics had an easy time painting her as either a liar or as someone who had been duped by an unscrupulous therapist.

Other individuals came forward with claims of having been ritually abused by satanic cults of adults who, they claimed, had murdered a large number of babies. Unfortunately, they had no reports of any missing children or forensic evidence they could point to that would back up their preposterous claims. Some unscrupulous psychiatrists got into the act and began to compare those who reported "recovered memories" with individuals who made obviously false claims of having been abducted by space aliens.

All of this led to the foundation of the False Memory Syndrome Foundation (FMSF), made up of parents of individuals who claimed to have been falsely accused by their grown children of episodes of child abuse when the accusers were young. The members and their patron saint, Elizabeth Loftus, seem to believe that most such claims are either outright lies or are made by victims of unscrupulous therapists, or even of self-help books such as *The Courage to Heal*. The argument that because some claims are fraudulent means therefore that most claims are fraudulent is an absurdity: the Piltdown Man argument once again.

In the vast majority of cases, seemingly "forgotten" memories of child abuse are triggered when people are *not* in psychotherapy. Often, the memories are the reasons why an individual *seeks* psychotherapy in the first place. Common triggers include environmental events that remind the victim of the earlier events, such as a TV news story about an abused child, or sometimes by what therapists call an "anniversary" reaction. A woman who was sexually abused by her father will suddenly "remember" the abuse when her daughter reaches the age when she, the mother, had been abused.

Of course, false accusations of abuse are sometimes made. Few studies have attempted to corroborate abuse claims in a large sample, although two investigations that did showed that most such accusations are probably true.[4,5] Many times a determination of the truth comes down to the word of the accused versus the word of the accuser, because there are no witnesses to the alleged child abuse. Particularly in the case of sexual abuse, abusers make sure that no witnesses come forward. They wait until they can get the child alone before proceeding. They also make sure that the child does not tell anyone, usually by issuing various threats. The child is warned that he or she will be removed from the family, that Daddy will not love him or her anymore, or that the abuser will kill him or her or other family members if he or she dares to tell anyone what happened.

To point out the obvious, someone being accused of child abuse has more motivation to lie than a child has to falsely claim victimization. As one pundit put it, maybe the FMSF should be renamed the False *Missing* Memories Syndrome Foundation. How do we know that some members of the FMSF are not pedophiles trying to cover their tracks? Sometimes the best defense is a good offense.

The people who believe that most "recovered" abuse accusations are false also conveniently ignore the fact that the whole Catholic Church sex abuse scandal started with a case of a recovered memory about a Catholic priest in Massachusetts, Father James Porter, by a man named Frank Fitzpatrick. Fitzpatrick's revelation of prolonged child sexual abuse by Father Porter led to an investigation that resulted in tape-recorded incriminatory statements by Porter, and eventual identification of dozens of his other victims. Porter was prosecuted criminally in Fall River, Massachusetts, and he pled guilty. A civil suit against the Catholic Church was settled on terms favorable to the plaintiffs, costing the church millions of dollars.

Critics of the concept of recovered memory point out that Fitzpatrick apparently later admitted that he had not really completely forgotten the trauma, but had merely pushed it out of his consciousness for many years. The question of whether or not repression is a valid concept can be, I believe, resolved with a slight alteration of the traditional conceptualization of repression. I believe that what Fitzpatrick experienced is the case in almost all instances of recovered memories. I believe that strict Freudian psychoanalysts were incorrect about the true nature of repressed memories. I believe instead that "pushing things out of one's consciousness" is, despite being somewhat of a conscious decision, the true definition of repression. If so-called "unconscious" memories were truly as irretrievable as some Freudians seem to believe, then they would never come back under any circumstances, including during psychoanalysis.

On what do I base this opinion? In over thirty years of clinical experience, none of my patients have ever unexpectedly "recovered" memories from their past during the later course of their psychotherapy. During my initial session, I take a fairly complete biographical history. Under the guise of "leaving no stone unturned," I nonchalantly ask them if they experienced any violence or abuse in their family as they grew up, and they almost always remember if they were abused or if they were not, although they may not share with me the true extent or scope of any abuse that had occurred. A few patients answer my initial inquiry about abuse by saying that they are uncertain if they have been abuse victims. These patients almost invariably admit later in treatment that their initial lack of certainty was due to a reluctance to think about their past.

Many patients, in fact, are absolutely certain that physical or sexual abuse did *not* occur, and these patients do not come up with "recovered" memories later in therapy. Any clear answer to my initial screening question almost invariably turns out to be the correct one. For my patients who say they were abused, I have not just taken their word for it. In cases where the abuse was perpetrated by family members, I have been frequently successful in coaching patients to use techniques that lead the abusers to confess to what they had done, although the confession may be somewhat indirect.

Sometimes my patients have related certain biographical information in the first session but then later deny ever having told it to me at all. One woman told me in our very first session that her father was an alcoholic. When I brought this up a few sessions later, she became angry and indignant and told me in no uncertain terms that she had said no such thing. Much later in therapy, I found out that there was some truth in both her initial description and her later denial. As it turned out, her father was not an alcoholic; he was a heroin addict. Rather than trying to paint their parents as abusive in order to blame the parents for the patients' own inadequacies, most victims of parental abuse are actually protective of their parents. Not only is exaggeration of the abuse rare, but in most instances it is instead *minimized.*

Another common quirk about memory is illustrated by many patients who report that they have *no* memories of anything that happened during their childhood between certain ages. However, if I ask them about, say, school experiences they had during that "forgotten" period without bringing up their previous statements about their amnesia, they can almost always tell me about events that took place during those years. Therefore, to say that they have no memory of those years whatsoever is not completely accurate.

Nonetheless, they do not seem to want to think about what went on then, and they act *as if* they have no recollection. They are not, therefore, actually lying. One fellow faculty member has opined that whenever his patients answer "I do not know" to a question about their past or about the reasons that they act in certain ways, they are really saying, "I do not want to think about it."

After a debate about repressed memory at an annual meeting of the APA during a question-and-answer period, I brought up the phenomenon of patients claiming to have global amnesia for certain periods of their lives. I asked the man who thought recovered memory was a hoax if he thought such patients were lying. Of note is that he completely sidestepped the question, much as abusive parents often do when confronted with the abuse. "You have to do a complete evaluation," he replied.

Of course I had done a complete evaluation of these patients; they had exhibited absolutely no evidence for any brain disorder that would lead to memory impairment. I did not get a chance to mention this and ask the man to actually answer the question I had asked. Over the years, I have seen a number of examples of "experts" sidestepping evidence that their assertions are problematic, or offering disingenuous counterarguments.

The Unreliability of Memory

Memory is a truly funny thing. A case in point is the so-called *Rashomon effect,* in which different people remember a series of events they all witnessed as a group in different and contradictory ways. A famous experiment, which has been replicated in countless college social psychology and law school classes, illustrates the phenomenon. During a lecture, a professor secretly arranges for several people to suddenly and unexpectedly descend on the lecture hall, do a bunch of crazy stuff, and then leave as suddenly as they had entered. The professor then has the students who observed the events write in detail about what they had seen. Almost every account turns out to be somewhat different, and in many cases markedly so. Some students were certain they had seen things that had actually not happened, while others missed fairly obvious events that had occurred.

We know that eyewitness testimony about crimes is often unreliable. Rape victims have been shown to frequently misidentify their assailants in police lineups. According to the Associated Press in a news article in August 2008, since 1991, 218 people were exonerated from rape through DNA testing, and in three-quarters of the cases, mistaken eyewitness identification was a major factor in the wrongful convictions.

Elizabeth Loftus points out that memory fades with time and becomes less accurate as original events become more distant. Memories can also be affected by what Loftus calls "post-event information." Witnesses are often exposed to information about particular occurrences from others who may be reporting hearsay or other types of misinformation. She conducted a study[6] in which subjects watched a film of a robbery involving a shooting and were then exposed to a television account of the event that contained erroneous details. When asked to recall what happened during the robbery, many subjects reported in detail false information from the television report instead of what actually happened in the original film, and vehemently believed in their new story even when asked if the news report may have influenced their memories.

A typical criticism of Loftus's work is that she does not take into account that traumatic events are thought to be processed by the brain differently than normal memories. However, a much larger issue that is raised by her ideas has only occasionally been addressed. Of course memories fade and become less reliable over time. Of course memories of specific details of events can be wrong. Of course memories of events that are witnessed for the very first time are subject to observer biases, missed aspects of the events, and sensory information that is misinterpreted. However, the big picture is unlikely to be misremembered. None of the subjects in Loftus's experiment confused the robbery they had witnessed on film with a film of someone taking an uneventful trip to the mall. One is highly unlikely to get being raped mixed up with having watched pornography on a computer.

Furthermore, identification of people or things being remembered becomes more accurate the more familiar those elements are to the observer. That should not come as a surprise to anyone who has an IQ higher than that of a stalk of celery, but at least one academic actually wasted his time doing a study that proved it.[7]

Crime victims whose assailants are strangers have only seen the assailant one time. Victims of incest usually live or have lived with their attackers and have been exposed to them countless times. Furthermore, child abuse takes place in a location in which only certain individuals ever make an appearance. If an assailant were a complete stranger to whom the victim had never been introduced—someone who is not *supposed to be where he or she is*—that fact would stand out rather conspicuously. It is extremely unlikely that someone being sexually abused would, for example, misidentify an intruder as her stepfather. She might not correctly remember what he was wearing at the time, how long it went on for, or even the dates that it happened, but those details are not especially important.

Even in cases in which individuals have always remembered recurring incidences of abuse by their parents during their childhood, some members of the FMSF and some of their supporters have accused them of relaying false memories. What makes this particularly reprehensible is that it recreates the *invalidation* that took place when the events were actually occurring. Victims of child abuse are essentially given the message "This never happened." The abused child must pretend that nothing is going on and that he or she is not upset about anything, all the while walking on eggshells lest he or she inadvertently reveal the abuse.

If the child does tell, say, the other parent right after the abuse takes place, not infrequently the other parent does not believe the story. Worse still, the victim may instead be blamed for causing the abuse. I have even seen cases in which the other parent actively collaborates with the abuser. The mother of one patient, after a particularly egregious and physically damaging act of sexual abuse by her father, immediately took the girl to a doctor and put her on birth control so her father could continue freely without impregnating her. The mother then gave the patient a copy of a novel about a little girl who was supposed to have been born evil. The role of invalidation in dysfunctional families will be discussed in detail later in this book.

Indelible Memories

Events that are emotionally salient, especially traumatic ones that have been repeated several times, are actually remembered more vividly and in more detail than other events because of the way in which the brain converts short-term memory into long-term memory. Contrary to a myth that many readers may have learned, the brain does not have a huge reserve of unused capacity. We now know that we actively use almost all of it. Routine events of little consequence are remembered for a short time, but then are pretty much forgotten forever. Most of us can remember our grade school teachers and certain things that they did, but what specifically went on in their classes on many unmemorable days pretty much escapes us. Events that make some sort of impression on us are far more likely to be remembered over the long term.

Studies are clear that short-term memory and long-term memory are different. One theory about dreaming is that REM sleep, during which most dreaming occurs, is the time during which short-term memories are converted by the brain into long-term memories. The reason dream content has so much emotional relevance is that emotion is used, in a sense, to mark information as either important or unimportant. The psychoanalysts talk about the "day residue" from which dreams spring. These are the events to which an emotional response had been elicited during the day and which are candidates for incorporation into long-term memory.

Despite the fact that traumatic memories are more vivid than other memories, individuals may still choose to avoid thinking about them. A study about victims of child sexual abuse in the *Journal of Consulting and Clinical Psychology* by Linda Meyer Williams[8] in December of 1994 that followed documented cases of child sexual abuse for seventeen years is often cited by those arguing in favor of the existence of repression. The study may seem to be at odds with the argument I just made.

These children, aged ten months to twelve years, were seen in hospital emergency rooms. Details of the abuse were recorded at the time of the visit. All of them showed clear evidence of sexual abuse. None of the reports were made in the context of a custody dispute, in which fabrication of instances of abuse by parents is more likely. Nonetheless, when interviewed seventeen years later, many of the victims said that they did not remember the abuse. One-third of those between ages seven and ten at the time of the hospital visit did not remember the abuse, and one-quarter of those aged eleven or twelve likewise did not recall it.

How is it that some of these children did not recall the incidents in question, when the events were so dramatic as to include a trip to a hospital? Did they "repress" them or just "forget" them? Again, certainty as to the answer to this question is completely impossible. Perhaps, once again, they did not want to think about the abuse, and so pushed it out of their conscious awareness.

The authors of the study argue that such is not the case because many of the women had no problems admitting to other embarrassing life events, including other incidents of abuse. Of note, however, is that those molested by strangers were more likely to report memories of the abuse than those molested by people they knew.

In addition, no information was collected in the hospital about the occurrence of previous incidents of sexual abuse or the number of other such incidents if any had occurred. We also do not know about important contextual elements, such as how various family members reacted when they became aware of the abuse, or whether it was kept hidden from important family members. The importance of contextual elements in determining the meaning of psychological phenomena will also be discussed later in this volume. Suffice it to say here that we cannot assess from this study whether or not the women had any particular possible motive for claiming that they did not recall the events in question, or for having pushed the memories out of their conscious awareness.

The usual explanation as to why certain memories are pushed out of awareness is that individuals are trying to avoid the pain associated with the memories. The affected individuals just cannot bear to think of how betrayed, angry, and helpless they felt at the hands of the very individuals who were supposed to love and protect them. Yet somehow most victims do recall the abuse. In fact, for many individuals, painful memories are almost impossible to forget. Sometimes the memories come into their heads as intrusive thoughts and images that the person cannot clear from his or her mind. This is one of the primary symptoms of posttraumatic stress disorder.

Studies have shown that the stress response in the neurological and endocrine (hormonal) systems of the brain can be significantly altered by ongoing child abuse.[9] Such changes may or may not be reversible given time, medication, and/or psychotherapy. Given ongoing traumas of approximately equal magnitude, some individuals may be more genetically vulnerable to such central nervous changes than others. This discrepancy may partially explain why some individuals are able to "forget" about the trauma while others cannot rid themselves of the memories.

However, I do not think this is the entire answer to the questions of differences in response patterns in abuse victims. One of the themes in my own work is that those individuals who claim to be unsure about memories of abuse when abuse actually had occurred—something far more common than the other way around—are not repressing the memories just to avoid pain and shame for themselves. I believe once again in the rather counterintuitive idea that they are unwilling to "tell on their families." In other words, they are protecting not just themselves but their families from shame. They are protecting the very people who abused them. We will later discuss why they would do such a thing. The notion that people protect their families will also provide a possible explanation for why individuals sometimes do make false accusations against their parents.

FALSE ACCUSATIONS OF ABUSE

While child abuse is most certainly fairly common, some accusations of child abuse are certainly false. In children, false accusations usually occur in the context of parental divorce proceedings, particularly if a nasty custody battle is taking place. The parent who has the most frequent contact with the child coaches the child to falsely accuse the other parent of abuse to help win total custody and deny visitation rights to the ex. Adults may also be asked to take sides by one of their parents against the other in a divorce proceeding, but adults are again not the same as children. They are not so easily swayed into perjuring themselves. Besides, most false abuse accusations made by adults do not occur in the context of a parental divorce.

One wonders how angry adults have to be at one or both of their parents to falsely accuse them of behavior as heinous as abusing a helpless child! Even if no abuse actually has taken place as claimed, I highly doubt that individuals who make such false claims come from relatively harmonious families of origin.

Such individuals may actually be *protecting* their families by *undermining their own credibility*. Having made obviously false or fanciful accusations, no one believes them when they tell the truth about what really went on in their families. They just may be proverbial CRY wolf. They may also in a sense be invalidating themselves, much as their parents may have invalidated them by falsely accusing them of having make up stories about abuse when they were younger.

An alternative explanation is that perhaps some individuals are highly suggestible and are vulnerable to overly zealous therapists who may have been abused themselves and who are therefore anxious to see abuse under every tree for the reasons previously discussed. We would then still have to ask, what *made* such individuals so suggestible that they would tarnish the image of their parents so thoroughly and cruelly? Were they born that way, with genes that determined that they would be suggestible?

Studies with hypnosis, a heightened state of suggestibility, indicate that almost no one can be hypnotized to do something that he or she would find morally reprehensible when not in a hypnotic state. I personally doubt that most adults who are not already justifiably angry at their parents can be induced by a therapist to falsely make such monstrous allegations. As we shall see, we are all very protective of our parents, even when on the surface we appear to be highly oppositional to them.

Patients who make absurd accusations against their parents in order to undermine their own credibility and cover up other parental misbehavior are not likely to admit to doing this to a therapist until they have formed a solid trusting relationship. Usually, they will not tell even then, unless the therapist specifically asks them about this possibility. Good therapists know how to ask such a question so as not to suggest to the patient the answer they have in mind.

Clues as to the possible existence of hidden reasons for making up abuse stories can be discerned in the description of an individual described in an article called "Cry Incest" by journalist Debbie Nathan in *Playboy* magazine in October 1992. The article describes a cultlike group therapy meeting for survivors of alleged sexual abuse. One of the women at the meeting was described as admitting that she had had no memories of sexual abuse. She was also quoted as saying that she was *ashamed* of this because she felt like she really did not fit into the group, having only suffered from emotional abuse. The pressure from the group and the group leader for her to "remember" sexual abuse was enormous and relentless.

The focus of the article was on the group leader and the pressure she and the rest of the group were putting on the woman to recall a supposedly repressed traumatic memory. In reading this, however, I was interested in the woman's behavior. Why should this woman feel ashamed of *not* having been sexually abused? Second, why, if she felt the way she did, had she come to the group meeting in the first place? If I were her therapist, I would have to find a nonthreatening and nonleading way to pose those questions if I truly wanted to understand her behavior and her feelings.

False claims can often easily be identified by a therapist because they contain a thinly disguised absurdity of some sort. At some level patients telling tall tales always know what is going on, even when they are caving in to pressure from a therapist. For example, one female patient who had been diagnosed with dissociative identity disorder, formerly called multiple personality disorder, questioned whether some of the memories that her former therapist had helped her to "recover" were accurate. The former therapist had told her that she had what she knew to be an impossibly high number of different personalities or *alters*. The therapist also had a negative reputation in town. The patient therefore assumed, quite reasonably, that she may have produced many of her "memories" of abuse at the therapist's behest. This did not change the fact that her childhood had been characterized by severe abuse. She and a sibling had, in a rare moment of working together, compared notes to try to arrive at the truth of what had actually taken place.

PARENT BASHING

Once again, bashing and blaming parents who have been abusive is not the answer to solving the emotional problems of disturbed and dysfunctional adults. As has been demonstrated time and time again, a cycle of abuse exists in which dysfunctional family patterns are transmitted from one generation to the next. Most abusive individuals were either abused as children or came from highly dysfunctional families. The grandparents likewise came from difficult backgrounds, and so forth back generation after generation. We might just as well get the blaming over with by assigning the fault entirely to Adam and Eve.

As in the case with guilty parents, blame is toxic in abuse cases because it often leads to an increase in abusive behavior rather than to a decrease. Blame is experienced as an attack on the personhood of the individual being subjected to it, rather than on just some of his or her behavior. It induces feelings of shame and guilt. Under such circumstances, the reaction of the troubled parent is likely to be one of fight or flight. The neglectful parent who is blamed withdraws, and the abusive parent who is blamed goes on the attack.

Another reason to avoid blaming parents is that, because of the cycle of abuse, abused and neglected individuals often learn to give as well as they get. They may psychologically abuse their parents as much or more than their parents have psychologically abused them. In a common example, elderly parents who try to make up for previous neglect or abuse are often told in a very nasty manner by their adult children that, in effect, their efforts are too little too late, and that they do not really mean it when they say they care. The offspring may engage in highly provocative or aggressive behavior, as we shall see when we discuss "spoiling," that in a sense allows the parents to say to others, "If you had a kid like that, you would have been abusive too."

The guilty parent phenomenon discussed in Chapter Two, in addition to fueling many of the public debates about child abuse, also provided fertile ground for the advancement of the financial interests of pharmaceutical companies and managed care insurance companies. Those entities started to push the idea that a medication is available that can solve almost every human problem. Neuroscience researchers, eager to advance their careers, twisted science in order to claim to have found biological and genetic causes for complex behavior problems. This is the subject of the next chapter.

4

It's a Disease! Psychiatry and Psychology Sell Out

Enter the drug companies looking for new mental disorders for which to sell pharmaceutical treatments, and looking to alter physician's medical prescribing practices. Although many new drugs are safer or better than older ones, profits are enormous if a majority of doctors can be convinced to prescribe expensive new brand-name medications instead of less expensive generic medications that may be equally or more effective and may have fewer or less dangerous side effects. Certainly it is better for big pharma if psychotherapy is not a patient's only treatment.

At the same time, economic pressures created by the rise of managed care insurance companies led practicing psychiatrists to spend less and less time with patients and to start looking for quick fixes for psychiatric complaints. The majority of today's psychiatrists limit their practice to writing prescriptions instead of employing time-consuming and less lucrative psychotherapy treatments. Statistics show that from 1996 through 2005, the percentage of visits to a psychiatrist involving psychotherapy fell from 44.4 to 28.9 percent, and the number of psychiatrists providing therapy for all of their patients fell from 19.1 to just 10.8 percent.[1] These numbers continue to fall. One patient of mine recently quoted a local psychiatrist as barking at him, "I don't want to hear about your mother and all that stuff. I just do meds!"

Meanwhile, clinical psychologists, who are therapists but not physicians, began to see their work devalued by the insurance companies on whom they were dependent for payment of their fees.

Their fees, along with those of every other mental health clinician, were ratcheted down. Fearing for their livelihoods, they began to prod state governments to allow them the privilege of prescribing psychiatric medications. For mental health practitioners of all sorts who continued to do psychotherapy, limits on the number of psychotherapy sessions that insurance companies would authorize led many of them to look for brief therapies for problems that may have been plaguing their patients for decades. For these patients, particularly those with major personality issues, brief therapy is often a complete waste of time.

This chapter will look critically at these phenomena. In the chapters that follow, we will look at some of the tricks of the trade of researchers who stack the deck to make genetic factors look more important than they really are, how a public emphasis on so-called "evidence-based medicine" has been used to tout highly flawed and manipulated data and to devalue more humanistic psychiatric and psychological interventions, and how all of these factors have led to a deterioration in the process of making accurate diagnoses of psychiatric disorders.

THE INFLUENCE OF BIG PHARMA

Major changes in pharmaceutical industry tactics for researching and marketing their products, beginning around 1980, created a fertile ground for both the industry and many academic psychiatrists to proclaim that almost all psychiatric disorders as well as common behavior problems are caused by genetically determined biological processes amenable to treatments with medications, rather than by all those nasty, complicated psychological and family problems that require psychotherapy treatment.

Since 1980, much of the research agenda in psychiatry as well as in other medical specialties has been hijacked by the pharmaceutical companies. In particular, much of the research has been severely limited to *clinical trials* of brand-name pharmacological agents. The operation of these studies is now dominated by individuals and companies with prominent motives other than the production of good science: a true conflict of interest.

The ways in which pharmaceutical companies have deceived both the public and the government, and the clear indications that these companies are often far more interested in their profits than in the truth about the effectiveness and side effects of their products, have been documented in several recent books, most importantly *The Truth about the Drug Companies*[2] by the former editor of the *New*

England Journal of Medicine, Marcia Angell. I will not repeat much of what is said in those books here, but will instead summarize some of the excesses that have specifically affected psychiatric practice in negative ways and that have furthered the devaluation of psychotherapy treatments that focus on family issues. Some of these marketing techniques are so insidious that psychiatrists are not even aware that they are being influenced.

I should mention that as of this writing many prominent people inside the government and academia have been speaking out against these abuses. Several academic institutions have now moved to curb the influence of pharmaceutical companies in medical education, and state and federal legislation is beginning to stop some of their most egregious excesses, such as the suppression of studies that show that their drugs are of questionable efficacy. However, much pseudo-science that is helpful in drug company marketing and profit making remains unchecked. Additionally, since this trend toward reform began, the least important of the corrupt practices have been the first to be eliminated. I will look at how individual studies are manipulated in Chapter Six. Here I will focus mostly on how pharmaceutical company influence operates on doctors through marketing techniques and involvement in psychiatric education.

Who Is Doing the Research?

Many people assume that potentially useful drugs are mostly discovered by scientists working for pharmaceutical companies, with perhaps some of the research being done by government-financed researchers in academic institutions such as medical schools or in the National Institutes of Health (NIH), which includes the National Institute of Mental Health (NIMH). After animal testing shows that a new compound is promising, independent academic researchers are then thought to run clinical studies to determine the safety and efficacy of the new medications in humans, again mostly with government funding or funding from the pharmaceutical companies.

The pro-business shift in the national mood in 1980 led to major changes in this process with the passage of the Bayh-Dole Act. This legislation allowed medical schools and universities to patent discoveries made with tax-supported research employing funds from the NIH and other sources. The schools could then license the new drugs to the pharmaceutical companies for marketing and distribution, and charge royalties. Later the NIH was allowed do this all by itself and make a profit. Thus, an unholy alliance between academic researchers and pharmaceutical companies was initiated.

Everyone involved could now make a lot of money when new drugs were sold more widely. Medical schools profited from the drug research that led to these lucrative patents. Research in psychology and psychotherapy took a back seat. In medical schools, faculty members could also procure more financing for drug research than for any other types of research. Most medical school faculty members are not paid by university or state funds, but have to bring in their own salary through research grants or through clinical practice. Therefore, their research must follow the money. Faculty physicians experienced tremendous pressure from administrators to focus almost exclusively on the type of funded research that might lead to a patent.

Drug companies became less involved with expensive basic research on new chemicals, because NIMH-funded academic researchers, along with small biotech firms, could do it for them. They also began to focus more on what Marcia Angell calls "me-too drugs" rather than innovative drugs for previously untreatable or poorly treatable illnesses. Me-too drugs are drugs that do the same thing as but are slightly different in chemical structure from another new drug that is hot on the market, and for which a separate patent can be obtained.

Me-too drugs can be extremely useful. For instance, there are six different brands of a kind of antidepressant medication know as selective serotonin reuptake inhibitors, or SSRIs for short, with more on the way. Each one has somewhat different side effects, and some patients respond much better to one of them than to another. Having a choice is useful for doctors since they have no way of knowing for certain in advance which agent will be best for which patient. Unfortunately, the profit-driven focus by pharmaceutical companies on developing me-too drugs diminishes research time spent on discovering novel agents for illnesses for which treatment options are more limited.

Pharmaceutical companies continue to control the testing on human research subjects necessary for obtaining approval from the Food and Drug Administration (FDA) for new drugs. They usually do this after they obtain the rights for the drug, to make certain that a new drug, should it pass the rigors of these clinical trials, belongs to them. Because of the profit motive, it is in the interest of companies to make sure that the trials are successful. The drug companies design their studies to stack the deck in favor of their new drugs, as will be described in later chapters. Negative studies that show a drug to be ineffective were, until recently, just not published or even deep-sixed. Studies with poor designs that did turn out to be favorable for the new drug were touted at medical meetings and distributed to working physicians by the ever-present pharmaceutical company salesperson known as the drug rep or detailer.

Many clinical trials are now done, not by academic scientists in universities, but by private for-profit groups known as contract research organizations (CRO). Science often takes a backseat to profit for these groups. They are paid by the drug companies on the basis of the number of appropriate research subjects they recruit. Therefore, overdiagnosing the psychiatric disorder being studied is in their financial interest, because having a higher number of subjects means more payments.

How CROs Bias Research Findings in Clinical Trials

Overdiagnosing a psychiatric disorder without appearing to do so is actually quite easy to do. The researchers who wish to do so can incorrectly use a standardized research interview designed for making psychiatric diagnoses on purpose. They use the diagnostic interview as more of a "symptom checklist," a subject on which I will have much more to say in Chapter Seven, rather than as a more thorough interview. This means they simply ask research subjects whether a symptom is present or absent and to rate its severity without checking to see if the subject really understands what the psychiatric symptom should look and feel like in order to be of diagnostic significance. Patients often describe perfectly normal emotions or behavior in their answers to a psychiatrist's questions about symptoms. These normal responses are then counted toward the required number of symptoms necessary to make a diagnosis, thereby increasing the number of subjects who seem to have the disorder being studied.

In a good psychiatric diagnostic interview, a doctor sometimes has to ask a question about a symptom in two or three different ways to get a meaningful response. The context and timing of when a symptom takes place also alter its diagnostic significance. If the doctor does not bother to ask about these factors and accepts any answer that the patient first gives, he or she may be misled. Just using a checklist in this manner does not cut the mustard.

If CRO doctors are still not getting a large enough number of subjects, they can further inflate their numbers by employing another trick that piggybacks on the symptom checklist ruse. They can accept at face value all "yes" answers from the patient to questions about symptoms, but if the patient answers "no," they can then probe further to see if they can find a way to get the patient to say something that they can interpret as indicating a "yes." In doing so, all ambiguous answers from the patient tend to be interpreted in the same direction. Conversely, to underdiagnose a condition, the doctor can probe the "yes" answers but not the "no" answers. As the computer folks say, garbage in, garbage out.

Still another way that studies can be biased is by mislabeling a drug's side effects as therapeutic effects. In a prime example, many very different emotional problems seem to "improve" if a patient becomes sedated on a drug and therefore appears less agitated. Because many new psychiatric drugs are sedating, nervous research subjects who are misdiagnosed may seem to improve on a medication anyway due solely to this side effect. These subjects are then mixed in with subjects who actually do have the disorder in question, who may or may not improve with sedation, and may or may not improve due to the actual therapeutic effects of the drug. The benefits of the drug in such a study may appear in the final results to be much greater than they actually are. Garbage in, garbage out.

Phony New Reasons to Take Medication

Getting back to the unholy alliance between academic researchers and pharmaceutical companies, the more a new drug sells after FDA approval, the happier everyone becomes. Several techniques are employed to artificially increase sales. One is to widen the range of patients to whom the drug can be sold by looking for several new *indications* or conditions for which the drug can be granted FDA approval.

In some cases existing generic drugs are just as effective as or even much better than the new drugs for these "new" indications. However, the older drugs have not been officially recognized or "approved" by the FDA for such indications because they were never subjected to clinical trials for that purpose by their original manufacturer. Once a drug is off patent, the company that first produced it has no incentive to pay for additional expensive clinical trials. The old drugs remain untested for the indication, although they may have already been widely used clinically for that purpose. The manufacturer of the new drug then makes the claim that its product is the only drug "recognized as effective by the FDA" for that indication in advertisements to doctors and sometimes to the public at large.

Another way to increase sales is to literally invent whole new diseases for which the drug is "effective." If a common problem like, say, being hypersensitive to criticism can be redefined as a biogenic disorder, voila! If the word gets out in just the right way, the financial stakeholders can have tens or maybe even hundreds of thousands of potential new customers who now "need" and clamor for their medication. Such treatment is jokingly referred to in some circles as "cosmetic psychopharmacology." Critics of the big pharmaceutical companies label attempts to change behavioral problems into mental disorders, as well as to change minor or vague physical maladies into diseases, as "disease mongering."

Starting in 1997, the FDA eased restrictions on direct to consumer (DTC) advertising of pharmaceutical agents on television, and the airwaves were soon filled with such commercials. In psychiatry, the commercials are often very effective in increasing sales because they help redefine and inflate the number of behavior problems that the average consumer believes can be helped with medication. The pharmaceutical companies brag that these ads are doing the public a service in that they are helping to "increase awareness" of these "conditions." Patients seeing the commercials then go to the psychiatrist and ask for the advertised medication by name, and the doctor will often comply after a cursory diagnostic interview.

Doctors do this, not only because they want their patients to think that they are accommodating, but also because they too often believe that the new drugs are better or that the patient has a brain disease instead of a behavior problem. Doctors, despite their protests to the contrary, are heavily influenced by the pharmaceutical companies because these companies also have heavily insinuated themselves into medical education in medical schools and residencies and into the continuing medical education (CME) required of practicing clinicians in order to maintain their state licenses.

Manipulating Psychiatric Education

The reader can appreciate how the content of medical education has been controlled and dominated by the pharmaceutical industry just from looking at a list of their activities. As already mentioned, many of the faculty members responsible for educating the next generation of psychiatrists are working on research that is funded by drug companies, but that may be just one of their many financial ties to big pharma.

Since the CROs are doing a lot of the clinical trials, many academics have started to earn extra income by giving "continuing medical education" talks, paid for by pharmaceutical companies, which are nothing more than thinly veiled advertisements for the companies' latest drugs. According to the *Wall Street Journal* Health

Blog of December 15, 2009, just one company (Pfizer) paid 3,700 U.S doctors $14.6 million in speaking and "consulting" fees in *one-quarter of one year.*

These "expert" academics go around the country as part of so-called *speakers' bureaus* for one or more companies. Psychiatrists and other physicians are enticed to listen to these talks with free meals at very expensive restaurants. For a while doctors could even bring their spouses along, although that practice was stopped by the pharma trade group after it was brought to public attention.

The speakers at these meetings employ a slide show that is prepared by the drug company, not by the speaker. The experts are not allowed to use their own slides, so what they say is almost completely controlled by the company. They are supposedly not allowed to discuss *off-label* or FDA nonapproved indications for a drug unless someone from the audience asks them about one, but they often do anyway. If such topics do arise from a question from the audience, regulations then allow them to say what they will. These speakers routinely minimize the side effects of the company's drug while talking extensively about the dangers of the side effects of any competitor's me-too drugs.

Generic drugs and psychotherapy are only briefly mentioned in these talks if they are mentioned at all. The speaker's prowess as a salesman is carefully monitored by the drug companies by checking to see if the doctors who attend the talks are writing more prescriptions for the new drugs. This information is easily available from local pharmacies. If the speaker is successful, he is given more opportunities to give the lucrative talks. These talks often earn far more money in a day for a doctor than can be made by treating patients.

For quite some time, many of these educational—I should say commercial—talks were presented at what were supposed to be scholarly presentations for medical schools called *grand rounds.* Because money for paying the fees and expenses required by many recognized experts to come to a school to present their research was becoming more scarce, departments of psychiatry would instead invite members of speakers' bureaus, whose way was paid by the drug companies. Thus, grand rounds became ground round.

Even lectures about seemingly nonpharmacological issues in the field have been brilliantly and cleverly turned into drug commercials. One striking example that sticks in my mind was a grand rounds presentation that was supposedly about medical malpractice in psychiatry. The first half of this talk actually was a fairly good discussion about what psychiatrists need to know about malpractice lawsuits and how to prevent them. The rest of the talk, however, was a warning about prescribing the antipsychotic drug Zyprexa because one of its very serious side effects was more common in that drug than in competing me-too drugs. If a patient were to develop this side effect, the speaker went on to say, he or she might sue the doctor for malpractice. The talk was sponsored by a company that manufactured one of Zyprexa's competitors.

Medical schools are beginning to curtail drug company commercials at grand rounds, but that does not mean doctors and trainees are no longer exposed to them. At the annual meeting of the APA, some of the presentations are designated as "Industry Sponsored Symposia." Plenty of other symposia, research papers, and other presentations are given at the convention that are not sponsored by commercial entities, but the industry-sponsored presentations are popular because they usually provide free meals for attendees.

Although supposedly reviewed by independent experts, the content of these symposia leans heavily toward advocating the use of certain drugs. Drug company funds are difficult for the APA to refuse because a significant part of the cost of putting on the whole convention is covered by the pharmaceutical industry. This is done in two ways: The APA is paid a tidy sum by the pharmaceutical company for the right to organize symposia, and it is also paid for space for huge commercial exhibits that are housed together in the convention center's main floor space.

Medical literature is by no means immune from drug company influence. Articles in journals are sometimes ghost-written by pharmaceutical companies rather than by the persons who supposedly did the research. Drug company advertising is widely seen in journals and in medical newspapers, as well as in so-called *throwaway journals* that are mailed free of charge to every psychiatrist in the country, and helps to keep the publications afloat. The publications sometimes do not wish to offend their benefactors by publishing articles critical of the companies' products. Articles in these journals have such helpful-sounding titles as "Emerging Therapies in the Treatment of Schizophrenia." The doctor reads the article thinking that doing so is a way to keep up with new developments in the field, but the so-called "new developments" turn out to be old news about the latest me-too brand-name drugs.

Even in reputable journals, articles touting off-label uses of medication are often prepared in advance by the marketing departments of drug companies, who then pay "experts" to add their names as authors even though the doctors may not have done any of the research themselves. This tactic was clearly demonstrated in a lawsuit against Pfizer by the U.S. Department of Justice over its marketing practices. According to the plea agreement that was posted on the Internet, some papers had no actual authors listed at all. Instead, the paper would say that the author was "to be determined" or "to be chosen."

Journal articles about research indicating possible new uses for old drugs, including uses that are not FDA approved, are given to practicing doctors, and until recently to residents, by the aforementioned drug reps. Drug reps seem to be chosen in many cases primarily for their ability to ingratiate themselves with physicians. Not uncommonly they are chosen for their good looks as well. I have dubbed some of them as "today's stewardesses." Not too long ago, all airline stewardesses were attractive females. Today's young female drug reps are usually, for want of a better term, hot. The men are not bad-looking either. These drug reps come bearing gifts: free samples of their medication so that unsuspecting patients can start developing brand-name allegiances, food, and until recently items such as pens or clocks that have a drug logo prominently placed on them.

As I mentioned earlier, efforts are being made to reduce the stranglehold of big pharma on medical education, but significant opposition from within the field remains. An example I witnessed was a talk given by Dr. Frederick Goodwin, former director of NIMH. Before this talk, he seemed to have decried the influence on the field of big pharma. He publicly bemoaned the fact that lithium, the drug of choice for bipolar or manic depressive disorder, was no longer being used very much as a firstline treatment.[3] Newer, less proven drugs like Depakote have been taking over the treatment of this disorder because of marketing efforts by their manufacturers, and many new residency graduates are no longer very familiar with lithium, which is much cheaper and less ridden with side effects.

Sometime after his views on this issue were published, Dr. Goodwin was scheduled to speak at a debate at an APA annual meeting over the influence of drug companies on psychiatric practice. I went to listen to the debate, fully expecting to hear Dr. Goodwin arguing in favor of efforts to reduce that influence. I was surprised to see him arguing for the other side. He argued vigorously that it was an insult to physicians to think that they could be so easily bought off with what he dismissed as "a pen and a pizza."

The marketing activities I described above go far beyond these little promotional gifts, so it seemed to me he was minimizing a problem that he himself had earlier described as being a major factor in the mistreatment of significant numbers of psychiatric patients.

I was puzzled to say the least. A possible clue to this mystery was published some years later in an article in the *New York Times* dated November 21, 2008. It stated that Dr. Goodwin had earned $1.3 million from 2000 to 2007 giving marketing lectures for pharmaceutical companies.

Reform That Is Barely Reform

Despite being relatively minor concerns, the pen and the pizza is what first got the attention of reformers. Pens with drug names imprinted on them are now a thing of the past. Detail folks have been banned from providing free lunches to residents by many medical schools. Though big pharma does like to develop relationships with doctors early in their training, this move may actually backfire. In the training program I led, reps had until recently been allowed to furnish lunch before a meeting or teaching seminar for the residents, and I allowed the reps to spend five to ten minutes promoting their products. They would then be asked to leave, and I would point out any statements they may have made that skewed the information they provided in favor of the drugs made by the company they represented.

For example, the reps may have presented a study that shows statistically that their drug is effective for a particular symptom. Later, I might have to point out that while the article showed results to be *statistically significant,* they were not *clinically significant.* Say, for example, that an antidepressant was shown in a study to reliably decrease the severity of a particular symptom in a significant percentage of patients, and the odds that this finding is just a coincidence are very small. However, if the drug decreases the symptom severity on average by only 2 percent, the drug is not of much benefit to patients. I guess it would be better than nothing, but not much.

Now that reps cannot come to talk to the residents at all, the first sustained exposure residents will have to the practices of pharmaceutical reps will take place after they enter practice. At that time, no faculty members will be around to provide them with a balanced view. Even when they are residents, however, doctors may continue to be influenced by drug reps, without balancing viewpoints, because residents are free to meet them at the many promotional dinners for practicing clinicians.

The marketing activities of the drug companies do not only revolve around expanding indications for their new and expensive drugs, but are also designed to denigrate drugs that have recently gone off-patent and are now available as cheaper generics. The goal is to decrease the sale of generics in favor of brand-name drugs that are in some cases actually less effective and more toxic than the newer drugs. In Chapters Six and Seven, we will see how this is taking place with the use of certain antidepressants, most of which have recently gone off patent, that are in actuality extremely good medications for many purposes.

Here I will discuss how pharmaceutical companies have helped to demonize some very effective but cheap medications called benzodiazepines that are very helpful in relieving common but debilitating anxiety due to life or relationship stress. I will spend a lot of time on this subject because it ties in to the trend of pathologizing, medicalizing, and misdiagnosing chronic anxiety as bipolar disorder, adult attention deficit hyperactivity disorder (ADHD), and other more serious mental disorders, which are then treated with potentially dangerous and expensive brand-name medications.

The argument is often made that if a symptom the patient shows can be treated with a medication that is effective for a certain disorder, then this is at least partial and indirect evidence that the patient has that disorder. In some situations this proposition may have some truth, but due to such factors as sedating side effects, in others it is sheer nonsense.

Benzodiazepines

Benzodiazepines are a group of tranquilizers that include such popular drugs as Valium, Librium, Klonopin, Ativan, Xanax, Dalmane, and Restoril. Most of the public, and many physicians who should know better, believe that some of these medications are tranquilizers, while others are sleeping pills. The truth is that they all do the same thing. They all operate on neurons that have a neurotransmitter called GABA. Neurotransmitters are the chemicals that are present between brain cells that allow different neurons to communicate with each other. Benzodiazepines all affect GABA levels in the brain in much the same way.

An old joke asks, "What is the difference between a tranquilizer and a sleeping pill?" The answer: marketing. This is the correct answer. All of the drugs help both anxiety and insomnia. The only major difference among them is important, however: They vary in terms of their *half-life,* the amount of time they stick around in the body before being eliminated. This is important because the shorter the half-life, the more addictive they are.

The sleeping pill versus tranquilizer issue leads to some very strange but nonetheless common prescribing practices. A patient is prescribed one benzodiazepine for anxiety, and a different one for sleep. This is silly because both problems could be solved with one medication. If the patient still has symptoms, this could be easily handled by either giving more of the medication at bedtime or by increasing the total dosage taken in a 24-hour period.

This issue of doctors prescribing one drug for anxiety and another for sleep has reached new highs of absurdity with the introduction of three "new" brand-name sleeping medications: Ambien, Lunesta, and Sonata. All three of these drugs are technically not benzodiazepines, but they might as well be. They have a slightly different chemical structure, but they do the same thing. They are called *nonbenzodiazepine benzodiazepine receptor agonists.* Loosely translated, this means that they affect the same nerve cells in exactly the same way as *benzodiazepine* benzodiazepine receptor agonists. They offer no advantage in terms of addictive potential, side effects, or efficacy. Anecdotally, many doctors do not seem to realize this. This is probably because they are marketed differently. Most benzos have been available generically for a long time, while the newer drugs have not.

To sell the new drugs, they were advertised as "new" and "different" without any specification of exactly how, and an army of pharmaceutical representatives and so-called "experts" fanned out to extol their use. DTC advertising for them was extremely heavy, so patients would demand them from their doctors. Ambien went generic not too long ago, so its distributor came out with a brand-name medication with the same active ingredient but a different formulation. It was a two-layer drug, one of which dissolved quickly and helped the patient get to sleep faster, while the other layer dissolved slowly so that sleep could be maintained throughout the night. That sounds good, but the exact same results can be obtained by using a benzo that is absorbed into the body quickly and has a long half-life. The most famous benzo of them all, Valium, does exactly that. If a person on Valium is too groggy upon awakening, this can be cured by lowering the dose.

Usage of benzodiazepines, when they were first introduced and were only available as brand-name drugs, quickly replaced the use of another class of drugs called barbiturates. This was a good thing. Barbiturates like Secanol or Nembutol are very dangerous drugs. They are far more addictive than benzos. Patients develop tolerance to them, meaning that they require higher and higher dosages to get the same effect. In most patients, benzos do not cause tolerance. Furthermore, barbiturates are extremely lethal in overdose, while a patient can take massive amounts of benzos and not die. While the combination of a benzo with alcohol can in rare instances be lethal, barbiturates plus alcohol is an exceptionally lethal combination.

While some people do abuse benzos, most patients who take them for anxiety or sleep, including former alcoholics,[4] do not abuse the medications. The individuals who do take higher doses of the drug than prescribed often do so because their doctors are so worried about addiction that the patients are not given a high enough dose of the medicine to control their symptoms. They take matters into their own hands. Still others become addicted because they are given very short-acting benzos like Xanax and experience withdrawal symptoms almost immediately if they miss a dose.

While stopping any benzo can produce withdrawal, tapering patients off of them slowly prevents it, and is extremely easy to do in any patient motivated to stop using them. Benzos do have street value, but on the street they are mostly used to cushion the "crash" when a user of amphetamines or cocaine comes down off of those drugs, as described in a song by Lou Reed, "Walk on the Wild Side."

Other than a very mild risk of dependence, benzos have virtually no side effects except in the very elderly. Almost no other class of drugs causes fewer problems. Still, the generic ones are now routinely denigrated in journals and psychiatric newspapers in ways that drugs like Lunesta are not. Since all of these medications are central nervous system depressants, they are said to cause or worsen depressive episodes in anyone prone to depression. After having observed their use in literally hundreds patients who were actively depressed or had a history of depression, I have never seen that happen, but maybe my experience is atypical. In the elderly, benzos can cause falls, slightly depress breathing in patients with chronic obstructive pulmonary disease, and increase memory impairment in individuals with mild memory difficulties to begin with. Some commentaries seem to imply that these are also reasons to avoid their use in young adults.

Benzos are extremely effective in patients with panic attacks, which are severe and debilitating anxiety attacks accompanied by an extensive set of highly unpleasant physical sensations and intense fear. However, for some reason SSRI antidepressants became the "treatment of choice" for panic attacks rather than benzos, although SSRIs tend to only reduce the frequency and severity of panic attacks and not stop them altogether. Benzos, alone or in combination with an SSRI, often do stop them cold. Furthermore, benzos effectively treat two types of anxiety seen in panic patients: the panic attack itself and the *anticipatory anxiety* created by the fear of having another attack. Anticipatory anxiety actually increases the likelihood of having another panic attack. SSRIs do not treat it.

SSRIs, while highly effective for treating clinical depression, obsessive-compulsive disorder, and some impulse control problems, also sometimes have more troublesome side effects than benzos. A big one is that they often tend to knock out patients' sex drive or impair sexual performance and satisfaction in both men and women. Which would you rather take if you had panic attacks, a more effective drug with a slight potential for addiction, or a less effective drug that took out your sex drive?

SSRIs have become the treatment of choice over benzos in panic disorder because, in my opinion, of the exaggeration by so-called experts in the field of the addictive potential and side effects of benzos in the years before most SSRIs went generic. When Valium was first released, it quickly became one of the most widely prescribed drugs in the world. Everyone seemed to be on it. In movie comedies, anyone becoming acutely anxious would immediately be surrounded by people generously offering a Valium from the bottles they themselves were apparently always carrying. Ever since almost all benzos went generic, however, more and more doctors began to refuse to prescribe them, for fear of causing addiction or some other unnamed harm.

Not surprisingly, some doctors and psychiatrists who hesitate to prescribe benzos seem to think drugs like Ambien are no problem at all, despite the fact that they are every bit as habit forming. These very same doctors may also have no problem prescribing far more dangerous drugs. The so-called *atypical* antipsychotic drugs are being prescribed more and more widely, even for sleep and anxiety. While very necessary for psychotic patients, these drugs can cause severe weight gain, high cholesterol, and sometimes diabetes. Again, would you rather risk becoming dependent on otherwise harmless benzos, or dependent on daily injections of insulin?

Additionally, some psychiatrists who are afraid of prescribing benzos hand out stimulants such as Adderall, an amphetamine, without a care. Even the Drug Enforcement Administration (DEA) recognizes that benzodiazepines have far less abuse potential than stimulants. Drugs of potential abuse are called *scheduled* drugs by the DEA, with lower schedule numbers meaning the drugs so listed cause more harm and more addiction than those with a higher number. Illegal drugs like heroin, thought to have no legitimate medical use, are on Schedule I. Stimulants and narcotics are both on Schedule II. Benzos are on Schedule IV.

WHY TREAT ANXIETY WHEN YOU CAN CALL IT
SOMETHING ELSE AND MAKE MORE MONEY?

What is going on here? In my opinion, benzos are being denigrated by the pharmaceutical companies and experts who are financially beholden to them because they are available as cheap generics. Of interest is that in a wide variety of journals, throwaway journals, and published treatment guidelines, whenever benzodiazepines are mentioned it seems that a phrase to the effect of "but of course they can cause dependence and addiction" is almost always added. When atypical antipsychotics are mentioned, in contradistinction, one almost never sees a phrase like "but of course these drugs can cause diabetes."

Also of interest is the fact that benzos were one of the few classes of medications that were completely banned from the new Medicare prescription drug benefit that was passed by Congress in December of 2003. The law was written so that some Medicaid recipients could not receive benzos as well.

The Medicare Prescription Drug Improvement and Modernization Act was clearly designed to maximize drug company profits at the expense of the public. This was obvious from the bill's absolute prohibition against allowing Medicare-contracted drug plans from using their size to bargain with the pharmaceutical companies for lower drug prices. The politicians pushing the bill did not even bother to concoct a lame rationalization for championing this provision. According to the *New York Times* of December 16, 2004, one of the congressmen shepherding the bill through the House of Representatives, a Louisiana Republican named Billy Tauzin, retired soon thereafter to take a $2 million job as president of the Pharmaceutical Research and Manufacturers of America (PhRMA). This is the main lobbying group for the drug companies.

Some commentators believe that PhRMA lobbyists practically wrote the bill. Whether this had anything to do with the banning of benzos is not clear, but anxiety is such a common problem that forcing doctors to prescribe more expensive medications for it would seem to be a good marketing move.

A second reason for the reduction in benzo use has to do with the trend of turning common anxiety into a brain disease. When doctors prescribe a benzodiazepine, they are often perceived by patients as treating only ordinary nervousness. Nothing wrong with that, but if doctors can instead prescribe something else for a more serious-sounding illness, they have a better rationalization for solely prescribing medications and not psychotherapy. They can say they are treating "diseases" such as "generalized anxiety disorder" or even "rapid cycling bipolar disorder" instead of anxiety.

When anxious patients respond to the sedating side effect of the drug, they may then be told that this is evidence that they have the disorder the doctor diagnosed them with. This type of specious reasoning has been surreptitiously applied in the overdiagnosis of bipolar disorder. It is correct that true mania is responsive to atypical antipsychotics—you know, the ones that can cause diabetes—and to some anti-epileptic drugs such as Depakote. If a chronically rambunctious and out-of-control child calms down and behaves himself after being given one of these drugs, this is taken as *prima facie* evidence that the child has bipolar disorder. This argument is made even if the boy does not show many of the other symptoms of bipolar disorder, or when clear psychosocial reasons for the child's behavior are present.

Almost all of these drugs can be very sedating. The higher the dose, the more sedating they are. They are all central nervous system depressants, just like benzodiazepines. Depakote even has similar effects on the neurotransmitter GABA that benzos have, although its mechanism of action is different and it is not habit forming. The behavior of the child described above may be due to anxiety and may therefore improve in studies only because of the side effects of the medications being used. I have yet to see a study in which these other drugs are compared for efficacy to a tranquilizer in this or many other populations, in order to rule this out as a possibility. I doubt that I ever will, because that would adversely affect the agenda of some pharmaceutical companies and some biological psychiatry researchers. I will have much more to say about bipolar disorder in Chapter Seven.

MANAGED CARE: PROFITS AHEAD OF PEOPLE

The trend toward medicalizing behavior problems has also been abetted by the financial shenanigans of insurance companies. Their avarice was given almost free rein in reaction to an economic difficulty experienced by big businesses and individuals alike: medical inflation. As most readers know, medical costs have risen much faster than general inflation. Since most medical insurance is paid for in the United States by employers, businesses have seen their expenses for medical insurance for their employees increase at an alarming rate. In some cases, the costs threaten their very survival.

Insurance companies were quick to jump into the fray and declare themselves the saviors of employers. They would "manage" the greed of doctors who allegedly enriched themselves by ordering too many treatments and keeping patients in the hospital too long, and thereby cut down the growth of health insurance premiums.

What happened, of course, is that managed care companies diverted money away from doctors and hospitals, who were the ones actually providing care for the patients, into their own pockets. Health care premiums continued to rise under managed care, but physicians' incomes eventually began to plateau. The profits of managed care firms and the salaries of their CEOs ate up a high percentage of insurance premiums. Literally millions of dollars were siphoned off. None of that money helped to take care of sick people.

Mental health took a particularly hard hit from managed care. In many cases, mental health benefits were *carved out of* or separated from general medical benefits and treated completely differently. Even though psychiatric problems are among the most common conditions in the general population and lead to incredible pain, dysfunction, and absenteeism from work, they do not tend to be as obvious or seem as dangerous to life and limb as general medical problems. Study after study show that the cost to employers from the psychiatric difficulties of employees in terms of worker absenteeism, disability, and job turnover is extremely high, yet many employers are willing to sacrifice mental health benefits to save money. Mental health problems are misunderstood and stigmatizing, and the effectiveness of good psychiatric treatment is not well known, so employees generally do not complain as much if their treatment options in mental health are limited compared to those for physical maladies.

Selling Them the Noose Used to Hang Us

In the days in which managed care first got started, the mental health profession was not helping its own case. Psychiatrists had a long history of hospitalizing patients who could have easily been treated in outpatient settings, and they kept patients in the hospital as long as they possibly could under the rationalization that more is better. Depressed or psychotic patients who were merely waiting for medication to kick in were treated with "occupational therapy" and "recreational therapy," which at times deserved their derisive reputation in the community as "basket weaving." The extensive misuse of psychiatric hospitals for acting-out adolescents has already been mentioned.

On the outpatient side, psychotherapy treatments in the psychoanalytic tradition were given to clients several times a week, often for years, with no clear-cut end point or consideration of efficacy.

Oftentimes the treatment seemed to be more for the "personal growth" of the individual in treatment than it was for treating a specific problem.

Managed care companies point to these former excesses and proudly brag that they helped to eliminate them, which in many ways they did, and I salute them for that. What they neglect to add is that they did not stop there. Where originally they had cut fat, they then cut muscle and bone. Hospital stays of severely impaired patients were cut to a few days, before many psychiatric treatments even have time to become effective, and suicidal patients were at times prematurely discharged with tragic results. Psychotherapy treatments were limited to a few sessions no matter how well ingrained or tenacious the dysfunctional behavior of the client was. Piles of paperwork were required of clinicians for reimbursement, the time-consuming completion of which cut into the time they spent with their patients.

For a physician like me to say that many managed care companies were incredibly dishonest and deceitful in finding ways to deny care and cheat physicians may seem self-serving, but unscrupulous insurance company tactics have been chronicled by many others with no such axe to grind. Their tactics are fairly well known. People in the general population hate managed care companies so much that insurance companies became the new villains in movies and television shows.

While certainly many of the people who work for them are well intentioned, as companies they are willing to let patients suffer or even die to increase their own profits, so long as employers do not drop their insurance products from benefits packages for employees. Their disingenuous rationalization for their behavior is that they do not dictate what treatments patients can get, only what treatments insurance will pay for. They certainly do not have to worry about being sued. No matter how egregious their denials of care, they were granted virtual immunity from lawsuits by the federal Employee Retirement Income Security Act of 1974 (ERISA).

I will focus here on just a few of their nefarious practices, the ones that led to the unfortunate predominance of the "med check" in psychiatry and ultra-short-term Band-Aid psychotherapy for major psychiatric and psychological problems.

How Managed Care Lied about How Much Psychotherapy Was Covered by Insurance

When managed care first took hold in mental health, many policies sold to employers and patients stated that twenty or more psychotherapy sessions per year were covered. This was highly deceptive because the companies would authorize only a small percentage of them as "medically necessary." They would then require therapists to waste hour upon hour getting authorization for additional sessions, which discouraged the clinician from even trying. Even if the therapist took the time, companies frequently denied that additional sessions were medically necessary. The therapist could then appeal the denial, but that would take significantly more additional unpaid hours of work.

The companies also used to have "gag orders" in the contracts that they furnished their providers, which are thankfully no longer allowed by law. These provisions mandated that doctors not tell patients about alternative, more expensive treatments that would help them more than the types of treatments the insurance company wanted to pay for. The insurance companies wanted patients to believe they were getting the best available treatment. Doctors were not supposed to tell patients that they thought that more treatment sessions were medically necessary than the number that the managed care company had authorized.

Another heinous practice occurred when the insurer's preferred provider panel changed for whatever reason. With next to no notice, severely damaged individuals would be torn away from therapists whom they had just started to trust and open up to. Months of patient work, in both senses of the word *patient*, would be completely undone. These patients, if they were courageous enough to even try, would have to start all over again with a new therapist.

Patients would also be discouraged from seeking help in the first place. One way this was accomplished was through the use of what has been termed the *phantom provider panel*. Only two or three clinicians were listed on an approved provider list, but a patient calling in was never able to get an appointment because they were always booked up. Alternately, potential patients might have to travel great distances to get to an approved clinician, and they sometimes just gave up on their desire to seek help.

In a way, the practice environment was better for both psychiatrists and nonmedical therapists in the days when insurance did not cover their services at all. Patients in those times came to treatment expecting to pay for therapy out of their own pockets. Under managed care, when patients do not feel better after having finished the number of sessions that their insurance companies tell them are medically necessary, even those who can afford it are often unwilling to pay for additional sessions. Some assume that all that can be done for them has already been done, so there is no point in continuing. That is precisely what the insurance company wants them to believe.

The companies had more tricks up their sleeves. For therapists who were naïve, unfamiliar with the psychotherapy literature, and not wise to corporate ways, managed care companies had several techniques for intimidating them so they would not request additional sessions beyond the small number authorized. When providers called the company to get authorization, they were made to feel incompetent because they had not been able to "cure" the client in six sessions. They were told that they were not up on the latest brief "solution-oriented" therapies. Alternatively, the therapist's integrity would be subtly maligned. The company voice on the other end of the phone would imply that the therapist was being dishonest about what the patient really needed because he or she wanted to make more money, just like those bad old therapists in the days when psychoanalysis was interminable.

Hassling psychotherapists over the number of sessions they would authorize eventually proved to be more expensive than just paying for the maximum, and rather low, number allowed by the patient's health plan. Approving the full complement of sessions also resulted in fewer complaints from employers that their employees were not happy with their health benefits. The insurance companies magnanimously stopped for the most part the practice of requiring frequent authorizations for outpatient treatment. Besides, they had, with the help of big pharma, academia, and other influences, already accomplished one of their highest-priority goals. A majority of psychiatrists had stopped doing psychotherapy altogether and concentrated instead on more lucrative and less time-consuming prescription writing.

Those psychiatrists that still thought therapy important hired psychologists or social workers to provide it for their patients, or referred their clientele to outside therapists in private practice. This was the birth of so-called *split treatment*. Some patients began to refer to the two different people managing their mental problems as "my psychopharmacologist" and "my therapist."

With some psychiatric conditions, split treatment has actually been shown to be less cost effective than having one person provide everything. To be successful, split treatment does require some coordination between the two providers, which eats up time. Having only one provider certainly prevents the problem that takes place when two clinicians work at cross-purposes because neither gets a complete picture of the patient, a situation that certain patients have a reputation for creating on purpose.

The Lost Art of Psychotherapy by Psychiatrists

In addition to avoiding the practice of psychotherapy because they made more money just writing prescriptions, many psychiatrists had already been completely suckered in by purveyors of the superiority of biological psychiatry. They began to be dismissive of psychosocial treatments in general. Many also wanted to be more accepted by the larger medical community, which had always considered psychiatry as a sort of stepchild, by becoming "real doctors" who focused only on the body. The specialty was in danger of being renamed "iatry," because the psyche was being taken clean out of it.

Many of these biology-obsessed psychiatrists were in highly influential positions in academic departments of psychiatry in medical schools. In some residency programs psychotherapy training was beginning to disappear altogether. In its place was a total emphasis, supposedly, on neuroscience. It was actually closer to a myopic view of one aspect of neuroscience rather than a complete view. The focus was almost entirely on neurotransmitters, those chemicals that allow one nerve cell to excite another nearby neuron, and the *receptor sites* on the second cell that received the different chemical signals.

The national body that accredits psychiatric residencies, the Residency Review Committee (RRC) section of the Accreditation Council for Graduate Medical Education (ACGME), became alarmed at the loss of psychotherapy training in residencies. The RRC consisted mostly of old-timers like me who believed that the focus on somatic treatments to the exclusion of psychological treatments was *reductionistic*. This means that this focus neglects the fact that a whole, such as a person, is far more than just the sum of its parts. Starting in July of 2002, the Psychiatry RRC mandated that residencies not only teach psychotherapy but also certify that their graduates are competent in several different types.

I was delighted. The forces in our medical school that would have pushed us to eliminate psychotherapy training from our program had to stop pushing us. Otherwise, they risked causing our program to lose its accreditation. A loss of the psychiatry residency would have adversely affected the whole medical school, because psychiatry is one of the departments that the body that accredits medical schools requires, and residents are often the primary teachers of medical students on ward rotations. Some of my training director counterparts at the more biological programs, however, were not at all happy to see the new mandates. I recall one training director at one mecca for biological psychiatry angrily wondering aloud, "What century is this anyway"? They thought molecular genetics was more important to psychiatry than thoughts and emotions, as if one could not study both.

Meanwhile, managed care companies had changed their tactics from requiring and then denying treatment authorizations to ratcheting down the fees of all mental health practitioners. The hourly rate many companies would pay for these services was an insult to anyone who had so many years of training after college. Psychotherapy as a treatment was once again hit the hardest, ensuring that many psychiatrists would feel that they could not afford to do psychotherapy even if they wanted to. Psychologists, whose incomes were threatened even more than those of psychiatrists, began to push for the right to prescribe medications themselves.

THE FIELD'S ANEMIC RESPONSE

If psychiatrists, psychologists, and social workers had stood up and refused to work for peanuts, the fees would have been forced back up to be more in line with the fees of other health care providers. Unfortunately, the federal government and the panic of the providers themselves combined to make sure that that never happened.

The insurance companies seemed to decrease fees in unison to very similar figures. I highly doubt that high-level communication about fees did not take place between them. Somehow, they were never accused by the Feds of antitrust violations. On the other hand, clinicians were warned that, if they attempted to join with other clinicians to set a standard for how much they were willing to work for, *they* would prosecuted for antitrust violations. I remember hearing that it was illegal for me to even ask other psychiatrists in my area what they were charging for various services. In a Kafkaesque move, Medicare administrators nonetheless expected me to know what the prevailing rates in my community were.

The fact that panicking psychologists were by then demanding the right to prescribe psychiatric medications set off a war between the APA and the American Psychological Association. Instead of standing together to fight for their rights and the rights of their patients, they went after each other. Some people referred to this fracas as an economic turf battle, but other important issues were involved.

Psychiatrists were starting to become in short supply, and psychologists argued that many patients had no access to medications at all. They would come to the rescue. Psychiatrists, on the other hand, know as physicians that psychiatric medications interact with all organ systems, not just the central nervous system, as well as with many nonpsychiatric medications and nonpsychiatric medical illnesses. Therefore, prescribers need to know about all of this, which means they need to go to medical school. Two of four military psychologists who had participated in training in one of the first pilot programs for psychologist prescribing privileges realized this and ended up doing just that. Still, the excesses of managed care should have been common ground for the two professions and taken precedence over the internecine dispute.

Many clinicians just rolled over and played dead, and this cowardice continues to this day. I recently received an e-mail on a psychotherapy research list-serve from a psychologist-in-training who seemed to me to be in grave danger of accepting the status quo by the time she entered practice. She wanted to know if there were intervention manuals for short-term psychotherapy for various diagnoses such as depression and anxiety. Some members of the list-serve gave her suggestions, which might under some circumstances be fine. However, the trainee also mentioned in her original e-mail that she was working in a "managed care medical setting where time-limited treatment is the only option."

In other words, if patients in that setting are more seriously disturbed and require longer and more intensive treatment, they are just plain out of luck. I knew that these patients would probably never be told this to their face, because then they might get angry or complain. I wrote back to the entire list-serve saying that providing treatment with this blanket limitation, and not being up-front about it with patients, is a bit like a group of cardiac surgeons saying to each other, "All we have to offer is single bypass surgery, but we will still tell patients that we will provide it for them even if they really need a double or a triple bypass."

The psychologist in training had unknowingly jumped aboard a bandwagon and wanted "evidence based treatments," the subject of Chapter Six, applicable for her work environment. I imagine that this line of thinking is encouraged there, but only so long as the evidence indicates that short-term psychotherapy is needed. When the evidence indicates that long-term treatment is more effective than short-term treatment for people with certain disorders, these companies suddenly do not wish to hear about it. Additionally, sometimes the "evidence" is inconclusive, cooked, or based on illogical inferences from the data, as we shall see.

HOW SOME PSYCHOTHERAPY EXPERTS ALSO ADDED FUEL TO THE FIRE

Some psychotherapists continue to tilt at windmills in search of short-term treatments that will appease their managed care tormentors. Many self-promoting psychotherapy gurus are ready to step in and provide them with ready-made "solutions." Some of these people are honest about what they are doing. They acknowledge that the psychotherapeutic measures that they recommend will only temporarily decrease some of the distressing symptoms and behavior for patients who really need longer-term therapy. They rationalize that people who have these symptoms are not going to be able to get the help that they really need anyway, so some help is better than no help at all.

Other gurus, however, made their reputations by proclaiming that their interventions produced miracle cures, such as helping cocaine addicts to stop using after two or three sessions. They based their outrageous and dubious claims on clinical anecdotes, a subject discussed in Chapter Six. In doing so they helped to give clinical anecdotes a bad name. Their clinical anecdotes certainly did not square with my clinical anecdotes.

Because human behavior is so strange and difficult to study and to change, psychotherapy has always been blessed with charismatic thinkers bearing new theories, techniques, and treatment paradigms for a variety of behavioral ills. In an explosion of creativity that lasted from the early 1970s through the 1990s, these people devised many new and ingenious techniques for influencing patients to change habitual maladaptive behavior. Their techniques were based on clinical observations and extensive experience. A "workshop circuit" grew across the United States for these leading lights to peddle their latest ideas to practicing therapists. To get clinicians to pay good money for these programs, workshop presenters had to be good showmen as well as innovative therapists.

I find nothing wrong in this proliferation of ideas. The proverbial cat can always be skinned in many different ways. When the exact same intervention is given to ten patients with a similar clinical presentation, the result is often ten altogether different and sometimes polar opposite responses. Give the same intervention to the same patient at different times, and completely different responses are also exhibited. Having many different arrows in one's quiver to draw from should any one of them fail is a necessity for successful psychotherapy.

As mentioned, however, some of these mavens strained credulity with their grandiose claims. The ludicrous nature of these claims was then used by critics with different axes to grind as ammunition with which to devalue the entire field of psychotherapy. While this was going on, those psychiatrists who bought into the brain disease model for everything behavioral, including relationship difficulties, had some new champions. Not only did they have clinical researchers with ties to big pharma on their side, but they were also seemingly validated by some basic neurobiology researchers. Some of these researchers unfortunately drew some illogical conclusions from their otherwise fine work.

I will here focus on one particularly bothersome type of statement that is made over and over again in studies employing new imaging technology that can study the structure and function of the human brain. In the next chapter, I will talk about deceptive tricks with which researchers strongly overemphasize the role of genes in determining human behavior.

NEUROIMAGING

Starting in the late 1970s, several different machines that could produce detailed images of the human brain in live subjects without surgical intervention or other harmful effects were invented. Some of these machines allow scientists to see which parts of the brain are the most active in living subjects who are engaged in various mental tasks or who show symptoms of psychiatric disorders. The technology behind these machines has continued to improve so that resolution has increased dramatically.

Examples of these machines include MRI, PET, SPECT, and fMRI scanners. Some use radioactive tracers that light up on an x-ray and that show structures as well as increased or decreased activity in certain parts of the brain. Others such as the MRI use magnetic fields. Since blood contains magnetic iron, the functional MRI (fMRI) machine has been particularly useful in visualizing changes in blood flow in different brain regions in real time. It can do this without the risks of using radioactive tracers. Psychiatric researchers and brain scientists have jumped on this new technology with fantastic results. For psychiatry, subjects with a given disorder are compared with subjects who do not have the disorder. Differences are often found, and this information tells us much we need to know about brain functioning.

While the results of these experiments are impressive, their interpretation can at times leave much to be desired. In particular, whenever the size or the activity level of certain parts of the brain shows these differences, especially in the more primitive, evolution-arily older part of the brain called the *limbic system*, the differences are immediately labeled as "abnormalities." Differences in limbic system structures may be due to some kind of disease, but they may not be. To automatically equate a difference with an abnormality in all cases is flat out illogical given what we now know about how brains work. Statements that imply this equivalency reflect either ignorance or willful disregard of the difference between *pathological* differences and *physiological* or normal differences.

A study[5] often cited by scientists who are critics of this sleight of hand best illustrates the point I am making. The study showed that London taxicab drivers have larger amounts of a type of brain tissue called *grey matter* in the posterior part of a limbic system structure called the *hippocampus* than do age-matched people from other occu-pations. Furthermore, the longer the cab driver has been driving, the bigger the difference. Using the difference-equals-abnormality line of reasoning, we would have to conclude that driving a London taxi is a disease.

Different parts of the brain light up when people solve puzzles or struggle with moral dilemmas compared to when they are not engaged in these tasks. This fact illustrates that all normal activities involve slightly different brain structures operating more or less at any given time, depending on the activity with which the person is engaged. Does this make struggling with moral dilemmas a disease?

We now know that the human brain is *plastic*. The more formal name for this is *neural plasticity*. Many brain structures not only light up differentially when they are active in a task, but they can actually change size depending on how much they are used. The brain has limited capacity and adjusts itself to environmental demands by recruiting for needed purposes neurons that would normally be engaged in other activities. For instance, the part of the brain that controls finger movements is considerably larger in concert violinists than in nonmusicians.[6] I suppose this means that being a concert violinist is also a disease.

Differences in brain structure and function that are observed in people with different emotional problems may not only be nonpath-ological, they may also be advantageous to the person's survival within the environment in which they operate. For example, the dif-ferences observed may be evidence of conditioned responses or adaptations to such circumstances as a chaotic family environment. Still, in article after article, observed differences are immediately labeled abnormalities. We will revisit this subject in Chapter Eight.

Also telling is that the so-called abnormalities that are observed on scans are useless in making a psychiatric diagnosis, so therefore these scans are not employed much in clinical psychiatric practice. The reasons for this are twofold. First, the differences may be due to only one attribute of the disorder under study rather than to the disorder per se. This particular attribute may be common to several other disorders.

For instance, brain differences may be caused by a patient's increased impulsivity rather than by a particular personality disorder. Impulsiveness is a trait shared by several different disorders. Attributes common to several different diagnoses are called *endophenotypes*. Often comparisons are made between sufferers of a particular disorder and those with no disorder, as opposed to sufferers of the other disorders that may overlap. When this occurs, differences in endophenotypes may be mislabeled as differences attributable to the full disorder.

Secondly, the scatter issue discussed in a previous chapter is certainly present in these studies. Although the *average* size of any brain structure may be larger in those with a particular disorder than it is in normal controls, some sufferers of the disorder may have structures that are considerably smaller than the average normal control. Conversely, a normal control may have a much larger structure than the average subject with the disorder. There is simply too much overlap between those who have and those who do not have the disorder to make the tests clinically useful.

Another commonly seen misinterpretation of the various differences found on brain scans is that they are evidence that some disorder or even some behavior is genetically determined. This of course completely ignores what we know about neural plasticity in response to environmental contingencies. If employed in the case of the London cabbies, this line of reasoning would lead to the absurd conclusion that the difference seen was due to genetic differences between the cabbies and the controls. For that to be true, genes would have to be a far more important determinant in one's job choice than they possibly could be. When human genes evolved, there were no vehicles to drive at all.

The literature on biological psychiatry and seminars given by researchers is rife with such logical errors and false "facts." I will be focusing on many more as we proceed. In the next chapter, I will start by discussing how genetic determinants of behavior are commonly exaggerated in the psychiatric literature and what good science actually shows.

5

The Heredity versus Environment Debate Revisited: What the Science Actually Says

Academic psychiatrists and psychologists often give lip service to the idea that the great debate in psychology over whether nature or nurture is more important in determining human behavior has been settled forever. It is said that both factors are always present, and that it is the *interaction* between genes and environment that determines the final outcome. There is some truth to this proposition, although it too is somewhat simplistic, but in debates between "biological" psychiatrists and psychotherapists, even this simplistic idea often goes straight out the window.

For a given behavior or behavioral syndrome, it is indeed true that genes, environmental influences, and their interaction are all invariably involved in one way or another. The question is, however, how much of each factor is operative? The answer to this question will be quite different depending on what behavior or disorder is being discussed. In casual debates, however, different behaviors and disorders may often be lumped together. Additionally, in human beings, there is a third major factor that is often left out of the debate entirely. It is a big one.

Human beings can think. This means that they can anticipate the consequences of their behavior and plan behavioral strategies to alter those consequences. They can formulate goals and then design tactics that are meant to achieve those goals. They also have motives, which determine which goals they choose to formulate. Environmental factors can alter their behavior, but people can alter their environment right back.

In this chapter I would like to revisit the heredity versus environment question to help readers understand how these various factors interact to produce behavioral outcomes in humans and to help them spot ways in which purveyors of various points of view mislead clinicians and the public into supporting their ideas. In particular, the influence of genes on behavior is routinely overstated, while the influence of social behavior is routinely underestimated.

DO GENES CODE FOR SPECIFIC BEHAVIOR?

According to Jim Medina, a neuroscientist who writes a column in the newspaper *Psychiatric Times* called "Molecules of the Mind," nonphysician neuroscientists mostly agree that the idea that one gene or one group of genes in higher organisms can dictate a specific complex behavior pattern is ludicrous. I agree. For one thing, there are simply not enough genes to code for the almost infinite variations seen in animal behavior.

Predicting what a brain will do based on its genetic structure alone is impossible because of neural plasticity. The brain does not function like a computer. A computer is hard-wired, meaning the connections in the circuitry do not change. In the brain, they change constantly. Ironically, even hard-wired computers at times do not do what they are supposed to. Readers who are familiar with the Microsoft Windows 98 operating system no doubt recall the infamous blue screen that could appear when commands from two programs unexpectedly conflicted with each other. The user would have to shut down and restart the whole machine for it to function again. Now try to imagine the predictability of a computer whose internal circuitry is constantly in flux.

Another consideration is that a system that rigidly dictated specific behavior would tend to disappear due to the evolutionary forces of natural selection. To survive under a wide variety of different environmental conditions and contingencies, the behavior of an organism must be somewhat flexible. If the organism cannot adapt to, say, the presence of a predator with different hunting habits, using a variety of different techniques to avoid capture depending on the exact environmental contingencies, then it would be picked off. Such organisms would likely not survive to reproduce in sufficient numbers to pass down their genes to the next generation.

Behavior that is completely determined by the genes that create the nervous system is called instinctual behavior. In mammals, almost all behavior of any complexity at all is not instinctual. There are of course exceptions, usually when there is some actual genetic defect, but they are fairly rare. In a contrasting example, a certain species of wasp can do a very complicated mating dance in front of a wasp of the opposite sex without ever having watched another wasp do the dance. The dance is done in exactly the same way by every individual wasp, and is done the same way each time it is performed by any given wasp. The behavior is wired into the wasp's nervous system.

Human beings, on the other hand, do not even know how to do something as basic to all of their biology as having sex in order to reproduce. The *urge* to have sex is instinctual, but exactly what behavior is involved, the naive human does not know. Someone either has to tell us, or we have to figure it out for ourselves through trial and error. Thankfully, most of us eventually get it right.

In other words, most of our behavior is either learned or planned. What genes do dictate is the *range* of options within which our behavior must fall. They limit the range of behaviors that are possible for the organism to perform. For this reason, all human behavior, from the most "normal" to the most pathological, has *some* level of genetic influence. Within the range, other factors come into play in determining what the animal actually does at a given moment in time.

Even within the range, of course, we all have natural genetic tendencies to react one way more often than another, but these tendencies can be overridden by conscious effort. Many of today's personality theorists posit three to five general factors to describe these tendencies in so-called normal individuals. For example, some people are more naturally extroverted, all other things being equal, while others tend to be more introverted. Nonetheless, even the most introverted person in the world can act like an extrovert in some environmental contexts. Unlike most neuroscientists, some biological psychiatrists seem to think that our behavior is completely determined by our genes.

Genes limit the structure of the human brain. They help fashion the connections between neurons and between different parts of the brain and determine which ones are possible to build. The building of the brain structures depends on the types of proteins and enzymes that can be produced by our genes, but also by the environmental circumstances under which genes are turned off and on. Therefore, whenever any type of behavior is studied, environmental factors will always be found to play some role, no matter how much influence the genes may also play.

The forms that human language can take illustrate the point I am trying to make. The linguist Noam Chomsky, one of the most

influential people in his field, made his name with the idea that
there is a "universal grammar" in humans that leads to a "language
organ" of sorts.[1] Our genetic endowment is what makes language
possible, and it limits the types of grammatical and syntactical forms
that are workable. Since a large variety of workable forms are available, many different languages can nonetheless be formed. Of
course, whether we speak Greek or Swahili is entirely determined
by our environment.

THE SOCIAL BRAIN

The genetic design of the human brain has been shaped through
the evolutionary forces of natural selection and by how well it functions in our natural environment. One of the activities that the brain
has been programmed most strongly to do is to *interact with other
human brains*. Human beings are among the most social of all organisms, and our survival has depended over our history on the survival of other members of our species, particular within our families
and our tribe. I will revisit this idea shortly when I discuss a concept
from the theory of evolution called *kin selection*.

The "gold standard" in determining whether any characteristic
of any animal is almost *entirely* genetic with minimal environmental
influence is something called the *monozygotic concordance rate* of
identical twins. The percentage of times within a research sample
that *both* of the two twins exhibit a certain characteristic is measured.
If two identical twins always show the same characteristic, then the
concordance rate is 100 percent, which means that the characteristic
in question can reasonably be assumed to be completely controlled
by the presence or absence of the same set of genes in both twins.

The concordance rate for almost every psychiatric condition,
even those known to have the highest genetic influence, is not
100 percent. In many cases, it is not even close to that.

CAUSES VERSUS RISK FACTORS

Almost no psychiatric conditions have a single specific "cause,"
either genetic or environmental, but rather have multiple possible
causes. These causes are better labeled as *risk factors*, because if present, each one makes it more or less *probable* that the condition will
manifest itself. When scientists study mental disorders, this fact is
often seemingly forgotten.

Other mistakes frequently seen in discussions of the data, in
addition to mistaking differences for abnormalities, are mistaking

effects for causes and mistaking correlation with causation. Does a difference in the size of a limbic system structure cause a disorder, or does the disorder lead to the difference in size? If the majority of heroin users drank beer before they became addicted, does that mean that drinking beer causes heroin addiction?

Published conclusions from research are sometimes as ludicrous as the proposition that headaches are caused by a deficiency in the human body of aspirin. Even the way different concepts are defined can lead to misleading conclusions. Some scientists themselves are confused about the issues I am about to discuss, while others knowingly create confusion in readers in order to shape scientific debates to their liking.

Necessary and Sufficient Causes

Before discussing the misuse of twin studies in psychiatry and psychology, I must first take a detour and examine the concepts of *necessary* and *sufficient* conditions in determining the etiology or cause of observed psychiatric phenomena. Even if the reader already understands these concepts, I would recommend reading this section. Necessary conditions are those factors in the absence of which a given phenomenon would never be produced. A sufficient condition is one in which, if the condition is present, the phenomenon would always be produced.

In the physical sciences, a condition may be necessary, sufficient, or both. For a billiard ball to move in a specific direction and go into a pocket, a certain amount of applied force is necessary, but the force might not be of sufficient direction, strength, and spin for the ball to actually get there. A force of a specified direction, strength, and spin may be sufficient to get the ball there, but might not be necessary, because another force of different dynamics can cause the ball to ricochet off the sides of the table in such a way that it would also go in the pocket.

In contrast, most psychological or psychiatric traits, symptoms, and disorders have *no necessary or sufficient causes*.[2] They have multiple risk factors, any combination of which may or may not produce the disorder. The more risk factors that are present, and the higher their magnitude, the *more likely* the psychological phenomenon will develop. However, for any single biological, psychological, or social risk factor, individuals will be found who have a lot of the risk factor but do not exhibit the entity in question. Conversely, individuals will always be found who have very little or none of the risk factor and floridly exhibit the entity.

To illustrate, allow me to use the issue of the relationship between a history of child sexual abuse and borderline personality disorder (BPD), a disorder that will be discussed in detail in Chapter Eight. Most studies have shown that among patients with the diagnosis, a good percentage of them had been victims of child sexual abuse. Nonetheless, most patients with the disorder have never been sexually abused, and most victims of childhood sexual abuse do not develop BPD.

The reason for the absence of necessary and sufficient conditions in almost all psychological phenomena is that the biological, psychological, and social environment in which people exist is so complex. No two individuals, no matter how close they are genetically or how much time they spend with one another, experience the universe during their existence in ways that are even remotely the same. I will elaborate on just a few aspects of the complexity involved.

First, almost all risk factors for psychological traits, disorders, and symptoms vary greatly on a continuum from very strong to very weak. Second, for each risk factor, several different mitigating factors also exist that, if present, can counterbalance the magnitude of the effect of the risk factor. For any given individual, any combination of the various possible mitigating factors and risk factors may or may not be present at any given time.

To complicate matters further, the mitigating factors also exist on a continuum from strong to weak. Third, the effects of both the risk factors and the mitigating factors that are present are independently altered by the frequency with which they occur and the length of time they are in play whenever they do occur. The final outcome is also affected by the issue of whether both a mitigating factor and a risk factor are present simultaneously, and how long a period they are both in play at the same time. Because of all of these influences, a phenomenon that scientists call chaos rears its ugly head. Small changes in the overall conditions, initially and at any time thereafter, can be magnified or dampened over time and by other influences and produce major changes in a final outcome.

Going back to the issue of child abuse, its effects are not determined solely by whether it is present or absent. Its magnitude or severity and its frequency are often cited as parameters that alter its effect, as well as the nature of the relationship between the victim and the perpetrator. Mitigating factors that are often cited include whether the nonabusive parent believes the child if the child tells him or her of the abuse, and if the other parent protects the child. Another mitigating factor is the presence of another sympathetic adult to whom the child can turn for help.

The situation is exponentially more complicated than even this. The effect of the abuse is influenced by far more than just these factors. Particularly in cases of incest, all aspects of the *whole* relationship between the child and both the abuser and the rest of the family over an extended period of time affect the final result. We all tend to "split" individuals into the categories "always abusive" or "never abusive" even though we all know that the abuse does not go on every minute of the day because the behavior is so reprehensible and defies understanding.

In point of fact, even the most abusive parent is nice and loving with the child on some occasions. Even while the abuse is occurring, its effect is also altered by other behavior transpiring at the same time. Some abusive fathers are warm and say nice things about their victims as they molest them. Others say mean things. Still others are nice and loving before the abuse and then say and do mean things afterwards. This latter condition may be the most difficult for the child because it is so confusing. A child cannot make sense of it.

Many mental health professionals do not seem to understand that necessary and sufficient causes or conditions do not exist for most psychiatric phenomena. Adding to the confusion, certain otherwise well-designed scientific studies can produce results that *seem* to indicate that a given "cause" is necessary, sufficient, neither, or both, but this result is nothing more than a statistical artifact.

Without getting too mathematical, most causative factors and presenting symptoms of psychiatric disorders are not constants. They are variables that exist on a continuum from mild or slight to severe. However, some studies have to simplify the situation by coding each cause and each effect categorically as either present or not present. In order to do this, the experimenter must dichotomize the variable under consideration by drawing a line indicating what level of severity or frequency is necessary for the variable to be counted as present. Depending on where the experimenters draw the two lines—one for the purported cause and one for the effect—the nature of the final outcome changes.

As an example with a potential cause, an experimenter must make a call on how abusive a parent needs to get before the child will be coded as having been abused. Does a light spanking count, or does the parent have to leave a bruise? As an example with an effect, how often does a patient have to exhibit unstable affect before that symptom is counted toward the diagnosis of BPD? If an experimenter draws the lines at one place, a cause may appear to be a necessary ingredient in producing the syndrome under study. If the lines are drawn at different places, this no longer appears to be the case.

Another way that scientists can spin the facts to make it appear that genetic factors are more important than they actually are in determining the causes of different psychiatric disorders is through the misleading use of the term *heritability*.

THE HERITABILITY FRAUD

Until the relatively recent discovery of laboratory techniques that have allowed us to map the human genome, direct observation of exactly which genes are present in those with a psychiatric disorder that are different from those without the disorder was not possible. To truly determine the genetic makeup of an individual and to sort out genetic effects from environmental ones, one has to know chemically what the structure of the DNA in his or her genes actually is.

DNA, as it turned out from the discoveries of Watson and Crick, is a very complex molecule that can literally have an almost infinite number of variations. Nonetheless, as many readers may know, it is only made up of four different building blocks. Each of these four smaller molecules is and can be paired with only one of the other three, and each pair is connected to another pair. The sequence of the pairs of molecules within a gene determines which proteins each gene codes for. Some of these proteins are used in the creation of body structures, while others are enzymes or catalysts that jumpstart certain chemical reactions.

Every cell in the body contains the genome for the entire body. In other words, all cells contain the blueprint for every other cell in the human body. Obviously, the vast majority of genes present in any given cell are turned off. Only the genes that code for the structure of the cell in question are active, and of those, only a minority are operating at any given time. Most genes are accompanied by adjacent DNA regions that are responsible for turning the genes off and on. A significant part of any strand of DNA contains these regions. Environmental influences travel by various physiological mechanisms to certain cells. Their arrival then initiates chemical reactions near the cell surface. These in turn start a chain reaction that leads to still other reactions within the cell nucleus that eventually produce chemicals that "sit" on the regulatory sites and either reactivate or resuppress a neighboring gene.

As mentioned, until recently, we could not directly observe this process. Scientists had to use other means to sort out genetic effects on people from environmental ones in studies for psychiatric conditions that did not demonstrate 100 percent concordance rates in identical twins. To understand how the term *heritability* is misused, let us first discuss how this has been done.

Twin Studies

Besides the measurement of monozygotic concordance rates, two other types of twin studies have provided the standard methods for this type of determination. First, identical twins, who have almost identical genomes, can be compared to fraternal twins, whose genomes are only as similar as those of any other pair of siblings. They are "almost" identical because postconception environmental effects can even alter this equivalency through the causation of mutations. Both identical and fraternal twins are presumed to have grown up in the same family environment, so researchers assume that any difference in the rates of any given psychiatric disorder between identical and fraternal twins reflects genetic differences.

The presumption of shared environments obviously is problematic, since no two people have identical environmental experiences, so environmental influences are divided up roughly into "shared" and "unshared" components. The determination of which environmental influences are shared and which are unshared has been extremely crude, but more on that later. If the concordance rate of a given characteristic or diagnosis is higher among identical twins than it is among fraternal twins, this may provide good evidence that a combination of genetic factors is operating. The bigger the difference, the stronger the genetic effects are. For reasons that will become clear shortly, the absolute value of the genetic component cannot be known just from these data.

A second type of twin study looks at identical twins who were raised apart from birth by different sets of parents. For cases to be the most instructive, one twin should be raised by the biological parents and the other by adoptive parents. In this situation, environmental factors, including genetic influences on the behavior of the people who are raising the twins, have been assumed to be different for the most part for each twin. If twins raised apart under such circumstances are equally prone to certain behaviors or behavioral disorders, then this finding might "prove" that genetic factors are paramount for those conditions rather than environmental ones. Most twin studies of this sort have been done in Scandinavia, where twin registries are most complete, in order to get enough pairs of twins raised apart to be meaningful from a statistical standpoint.

Studies of this sort have shown that alcoholism, to cite a commonly used example, seems to have a very strong genetic component. Whether or not adoptive parents are alcoholic seemingly has less effect on whether or not the twins turn out to be alcoholics themselves than the status of the biological parents. In these studies, if the biological parents are alcoholics, the alcoholism rate in the twin raised by the adoptive parents is still high and very close to the rate in the twin raised by the biological parents.

The True Definition of Heritability

Studies using these designs are used to arrive at a statistic called "heritability." The term is derived from the word *inherited*. One can inherit something through biological genetics, but one can also inherit something through nonbiological means, such as by being left money in a will. In fact, this double meaning is, literally, incorporated into what should be meant by the term *heritable*. Nonetheless, the term *heritable* is generally used in psychiatry and psychology journals to mean only genetic. *Heritable* and *genetic* are not synonyms.

The statistic derived from twin studies is not a measure of *genotype* but of *phenotype*. Genotype is to the actual sequence of molecule pairs in the DNA of which an individual's genes are made. As mentioned, we have only recently been able to directly measure genotype. Phenotype, on the other hand, is the final result of the interaction between the gene and the environment. Most of the genes in a cell, even the ones that are at times active in a given type of cell such as a neuron, are in the "off position" most of the time. They are inactive.

To illustrate better how this affects the heritability statistic, let us say that a man is genetically prone to be, all other things being equal, extroverted. Let us further suppose that the parents of said man beat him mercilessly every time he was exuberant. Most likely, such a person as an adult would turn out not to be *as* extroverted, on the average, as someone with a similar genome who did not have this experience. The end result—how extroverted the person was on average—is what is being measured in a twin study. His level of extroversion would be determined by the genes *plus* a gene-environment *interactional* component. The heritability statistic, a measure of phenotype, is exactly that: a statistic that combines purely genetic effects with a gene-environmental interaction effect. To call heritability a measure of purely genetic components is a complete fabrication.

Some may argue that it is at least a rough estimate of purely genetic influences. In some cases, it may be. However, the genetic-environmental interaction component of the heritability statistic can vary widely and can also be quite substantial. This is shown by just one fact alone: heritability for a given trait is never a constant in a given population but changes with external circumstances. This occurs even when a disease is already known to be completely genetic in origin.

For example, the disease phenylketonuria is solely caused by a bad gene that leads to a deficiency of an enzyme necessary to metabolize certain proteins. If a sufferer sticks to a specific diet, however, the disease "disappears" in his or her phenotype. If heritability were by some quirk of fate unknowingly measured in a population of twin children who had stuck to the diet since birth, who were classified as having the disease only if they had ever become sick after eating, and were known to have parents who have the disease, the heritability of this disease, caused solely by a defective gene, would appear to be zero!

Fonagy et al.[3] suggested the characteristic of human height as another example of how substantial the contribution of gene-environmental interaction effects can be in heritability. Average human height is determined both by genetic influences and by certain environmental influences like diet. Studies of the heritability of human height have shown different results in different populations, but it is approximately 80 percent. Does this mean that height is determined 20 percent by things like diet and 80 percent by genes?

No! To understand why not, consider that if a heritability study had been performed on a particular population 100 years ago, the heritability of human height most likely would have turned out to be about the same in that population as it is today. Although this type of study was not being done then, luckily the Czech Republic has kept some relevant statistics.[4] We know that the average thirteen-year-old boy in today's Czech Republic is fully 7.5 inches taller than the average thirteen-year-old Czech boy about 100 years ago. Since I know of no history of selective breeding for tallness in that country, one must assume that the Czech gene pool for height has not changed significantly over the last century, only the diet and other environmental factors. Seven inches is a very significant percentage of total height. In this case, the phenotypic characteristic changed significantly with no change in either the heritability *or* the genome because of a *cohort effect*. Today's worst diets are probably better than some of the better diets back then.

To see how this relates to behavioral disorders, we have to factor in that the social behavior within a family is a major environmental influence on the behavior of both children and parents. Let us look at how a gene-interaction effect might inflate the heritability statistic in behavior studies and how that would be quite misleading if *heritability* were used as a synonym for *genetic*. Let us say that an adoptive mother of a young baby has low self-esteem and is highly anxious and unsure of her parenting skills. Let us assume further that she has a relatively short fuse.

As most parents know, a genetically colicky baby is a lot more difficult to take care of than one with genes that lead it to have a very mellow disposition. The former child would be more troublesome to our hypothetical mother, who might respond in negative ways that might rarely occur if the baby were quiet, such as by becoming verbally abusive. If the mother's negative behavior occurred frequently, this could have an adverse affect on the future behavior of the child.

In a sense, the baby's genotype can *draw out* certain behavior from its caretakers that might affect its phenotype in ways that might not be seen if the baby had a different genotype. This would be an example of a gene-environmental interaction contribution to heritability. The degree and frequency of the negative behavior from the mother elicited by the child's colic would also be determined in part by the *mother's* phenotype, which also has a genetic component as well as a gene-environmental interaction component. The heritability of the trait of being temperamental in twin children of temperamental parents, raised apart, would be larger than purely genetic effects simply because the behavior of the child *helps to create* an environment that is similar for both of them.

Another way that the heritability statistic can be misleading has to do with the mathematics behind the phenomenon of necessary and sufficient causation discussed in the last section. The final heritability number can be manipulated in a study of twins by how high a bar is set for saying a given characteristic is present or absent. Let us go back to alcoholism. How much does a person have to drink in order to be an alcoholic?

If the designers of a twin study set the bar very, very low, they will of course find a lot more alcoholics in their entire subject population than if they set it extremely high. If the bar is set low, the concordance rate for alcoholism of identical twins raised apart will be artificially elevated, because the odds are very good that both twins will do some level of drinking, which may or may not be significant in their particular cases. This will then inflate the level of heritability found in the study. If the bar is set too high, the heritability level will also appear to change. The heritability level is in fact affected in one direction or the other by *wherever* the bar is set. If scientists are out to prove that alcoholism is or is not primarily genetic, they may be tempted to set the bar accordingly.

MORE ON GENE-ENVIRONMENT INTERACTION

This interplay between genes and environment was demonstrated beautifully in a study by Avshalom Caspi and others that was reported in the journal *Science* in August 2002.[5] Their results have been replicated in some other studies but not in all of them, so they have to be interpreted with some caution, but they are striking. This study looked at correlations between two different versions of a particular gene that produces an enzyme called MAOA and the level of violent behavior in children. The children in the study were actually subjected to genotyping; the study was not based solely on phenotype.

Lower levels of MAOA are linked with aggression in humans. One of the two forms of the gene that produces it is linked with a lower level of the enzyme than the other. In families where there was no maltreatment of the children, the difference in the level of measured violent behavior over time between those children with the "good" and the "bad" gene was fairly small. In families in which maltreatment was severe, the results were very different.

In the latter case, kids with the good gene showed a level of violence that was significantly higher than either of the groups of nonmaltreated children. If the mistreated child had the bad gene, however, the level of violence really skyrocketed compared to all three of the other groups. A similar pattern was observed in the relationship between the different versions of MAOA, childhood sexual abuse, and the later development of alcoholism and antisocial traits in females.[6]

Another experiment clearly shows the importance of social context in determining how brains of primates operate in the natural environment.[7] As discussed by Leslie Brothers in her book, *Friday's Footprint*, a certain type of brain injury inflicted on members of some species of monkeys led to one type of behavior when the animals were caged but to the opposite behavior when they were out in the wild with their brethren. The caged animals became tame, put inappropriate objects in their mouths, and attempted to mate with anything nearby, even animals from different species. Out in the wild, they never put objects in their mouths, were not hypersexual, were extremely fearful of even members of their own species, and eventually isolated themselves. The results of the very same brain lesion depended completely, not only on the animal's individual genetic makeup, but also on the social environment of the afflicted individual.

The brains of primates, and most likely humans as well, have specific cells, called "mirror neurons," that react to the behavior of other individuals in the environment. These neurons fire when an animal performs certain actions, but they also fire in an identical manner when the animal observes another animal performing the same action, as if the animal itself was performing it. Mirror neurons may function in helping individuals learn by watching other individuals model certain behavior. Learning through modeling is a prime focus of a theory in psychology called social learning theory. Mirror neurons may also be involved in our ability to empathize with others.

In teasing out environmental versus genetic effects in twin studies, I earlier mentioned the issue of shared versus unshared environmental influences. I now turn to that issue.

THE SHARED AND THE UNSHARED

I earlier alluded to the fact that investigators doing heritability studies of siblings divide environmental influences on them into shared and unshared influences. Shared influences are those presumably experienced by both members of a sibling pair, while unshared influences are not. In actuality, a determination of which parts of their environment are shared and which are unshared has a lot in common with finding water with a divining rod. Just because two children are close in age and grew up in the same household does not mean that they had even remotely similar experiences.

Unbelievably, I still occasionally hear the argument that a particular behavioral disorder could not possibly be shaped primarily by dysfunctional relationships with parents, because siblings of the offending parents have turned out so differently. That siblings turn out differently is quite true. In fact, they can and often do turn out to be polar opposites. In some families, for example, one son becomes a workaholic and the other a lazy freeloader who refuses to keep a job. I have difficulty imagining a genetic mechanism that would lead to an outcome like that, but it can be easily explained by looking at family dynamics and psychology.

The Smothers Brothers comedy duo made an entire career out of feigned sibling rivalry, summed up by Tommy Smother's catch phrase, "Ma always liked you best." Clearly this theme resonated with a lot of people. Do any parents really treat all of their children in a nearly identical manner? How could they? Children are born with major differences from one another that force parents to react differently even if they try not to. Even more important, anyone who thinks that some parents do not pick out some of their children to treat like Cinderellas and others to treat like princesses has his or her head in the sand.

In some ethnic groups, contrasting and seemingly unfair treatment of siblings because of their birth order is actually mandated by the culture. For example, in some Chinese families the oldest son often is groomed to inherit the family business, while a younger brother inherits much less if anything. In many Mexican American families, the oldest daughter has the duty to look after her younger siblings. She may have to forego her own high school social life in order to do so, while her younger sister has far fewer family obligations and gets to party on. Of course, parental behavior is not the only influence on how children turn out after they grow up, but it remains one of the most important ones.

SOCIAL LEARNING AND THE BRAIN

How does a fixed complement of genes allow for behavioral flexibility in mammals under a wide variety of unpredictable and perhaps never-before-encountered environmental contingencies? Scientists are beginning to understand how this happens. I previously mentioned neural plasticity. That term not only applies to the way neurons can be recruited by different parts of the brain to help in functions that they were not originally intended to perform, but also to the way that synaptic connections can form, strengthen, weaken, or be lost altogether.

These connections help brain cells to communicate with one another and form the neural networks that are responsible for all behavior from fight or flight to memory to moral reasoning. Each neuron in the brain is connected to hundreds of different neurons; some of these connections in the same cell are very active and some connections are less so. The total number of connections in the brain is over 1 trillion.

When a part of the brain lights up in a scan during a particular activity, that only indicates that more of the synapses are active in that part of the brain than before, not that they all are. In order to understand brain functioning, some biological psychiatrists have focused almost exclusively on the different neurotransmitters present between cells in parts of the brain that are active during a particular task. This tells us nothing about why some particular synapses in some neural networks in that part of the brain are active at a particular time and why others are not. Certain neurotransmitters may seem at first to be the only ones involved in a particular activity, but further research usually indicates that many others are also involved. Some scientists seem to develop myopia based on the earlier findings.

A good example of this is the neurobiology of schizophrenia. For decades people studying this disorder focused on a neurotransmitter called dopamine. Now we know that dopamine levels in schizophrenia are regulated by several other neurotransmitters such as glutamate. Almost all of the neurotransmitters we know of, and there are quite a few, are ubiquitous in the brain, and they are all involved in intricate feedback loops. While they are of utmost importance in allowing nerve cells to communicate with one another the way they should, they are not as important in determining which particular synaptic pathways are activated at a given time, particularly in areas of the brain that are important in responding to social and environmental contingencies.

Neuronal connections are constantly changing even from conception. Studies have shown that the migration of neurons to form the brain in utero is completely different for each individual, even for identical twins. One of the most important determinants of which synapses form, become stronger, become weaker, or disappear after birth is learning. Social learning is especially powerful in leading to these changes.

Long-Term Potentiation and Social Learning

An increase in the strength of a synapse occurs through a process called *long-term potentiation*. What this means in a nutshell is that stimulating a synapse once or twice only leads to short-term changes in its strength, which then disappear. When a synapse is stimulated more than that, however, new proteins are produced in the neuron on the receiving end of the synapse that lead to a more permanent increase in strength. This strengthening happens not only in the one synapse but also in other nearby synapses.[8]

Certain areas of the brain are important in serving as a sort of early warning and response center for the brain to both danger signals and to important social signals. These areas are called the amygdala, the anterior cingulate gyrus, and the orbital frontal cortex. Neural pathways that encode early patterns of social attachment, social stimulus appraisal (*social cognition*), and fight or flight responses to fear are all centered in these areas.[9] Damage to the amygdala in monkeys leads to impairment in their ability to respond appropriately to the approach of other monkeys.[10] Monkeys thusly impaired cannot tell whether another monkey is coming to attack them or to mate with them.

Responding quickly to both environmental dangers and social cues has important survival value. If we had to stop and think each time we were confronted with commonly encountered situations, we would be nearly paralyzed. Therefore, much of our habitual behavior in social situations as well as our fight or flight response to fears is set in motion by the neural pathways in these brain areas. The thinking parts of the brain can override the initial response, but they do not kick in until after the habitual responses are first triggered.

The Importance of Attachment Figures

Attachment research indicates that these same regions of the brain use input from the emotional states of attachment figures such as parents to regulate both internal and external responses and emotions. Amygdala activities, for example, include both face recognition and initiation of fight or flight. Certain neurons respond only to certain facial features like noses, while others only to specific faces.[11]

Entire reactive behavioral sequences, which are learned early in life, are specifically reactive to each important individual within a person's family. Problematic reactions can be seen to occur with one parent but not the other. These reactions can be set off later in life by environmental conditions that mimic those experienced early in life. This may be the neurobiological mechanism for transference reactions.

Early learning may be particularly difficult to inhibit. The early fear tracks are not as plastic as are other tracks in the brain. They never really go away, although they can be overridden by newly formed neural pathways.[12] In general, it is much harder to unlearn fear than to learn it in the first place, a fact highly consistent with the experience of psychotherapists trying to extinguish chronic anxiety, particularly chronic interpersonal anxiety.

The suppression of fear responses has also been found to be context specific. If a fear response is weakened in one context, it may come right back if an animal is moved to a different environment that is similar to the one in which the fear originated. In particular, if the new environment is similar to the early family environment, fearful patterns of behavior learned early in life but inappropriate for the new environment may often be seen.

Because of these processes, early attachment figures may be the most potent environmental influences of all on our social behavior throughout most of our lives. For this reason, almost all forms of psychotherapy at one time or another focus on a patient's relationship with his or her parents, as we shall see in Chapter Nine. The power of parental influence over our social behavior does not diminish dramatically as we get older, although it does decrease somewhat.

Parents do not necessarily want to wield this sort of power. Their actions, including their verbal behavior, have a lightning-fast effect on us even if they try very hard not to have any effect on us at all, or even if they try to push us away. We do not have to see them very often for this to occur. We have a sort of tape recording of them that we carry around in our heads. My parents have been deceased for decades, but as I proceed in doing something about which they might disapprove, I still have a strange feeling about it. Many of us find ourselves saying things to our own children that were said to us by our parents, despite the fact that we once vowed to ourselves that we would never do that. When people return to their parents' home after a long absence, many of them immediately feel like they are adolescents once again.

WHAT OTHER DISCIPLINES TELL US ABOUT THE POWER OF THE SOCIAL ENVIRONMENT TO SHAPE HUMAN BEHAVIOR

Advocates for purely pharmacological approaches for the treatment of almost any psychological problem and for the proposition that genetics is more important than environment in determining behavior usually avoid mentioning or even reading studies from other fields that might lead them to question this proposition. The most egregious example is the neglect of a large body of powerful and well-designed studies from social psychology. In all fairness, hyperbiological psychiatrists are not the only ones that ignore social psychology. Many theorists from certain psychotherapy schools also remain blissfully ignorant of it.

An extremely important contribution of social psychology is the quite obvious observation that people behave very differently when in groups than they do when they are alone or with one or two other persons. Social psychologists have demonstrated time and time again that, given the right social environmental conditions, a high percentage of individuals can be induced to behave in just about any conceivable way. This can be seen most easily by looking at admittedly very extreme examples, such as the behavior of people in cults.

Now I understand that only certain types of people are attracted to cults. Their proneness to doing so may have genetic influences, but how much we do not know. Cult members are undoubtedly composed of individuals with a wide variety of different genes that make them prone to do a lot of different things. There is no evidence that people who are attracted to cults also are more genetically prone to suicide, so the following two examples are instructive.

In Jonestown, Guyana, in November 1978, 918 cult members died at the behest of the cult leader, Jim Jones. Although many may have been murdered, the majority of them willingly killed themselves with poisoned Flavor Aid. By all accounts, before going to Guyana, most of these individuals appeared to be happy and non-suicidal. In 1997, 38 members of the Heaven's Gate cult also committed mass suicide, believing that they would be picked up by a passing comet. Again, there is no evidence that this cult was composed of psychotic individuals who were delusional. We do not know, of course, if they had suicidal tendencies before entering the cult, but I can think of no obvious reason to think that they did.

I will briefly mention three famous early studies from social psychology that dramatically illustrate the power of social influence. Solomon Asch[13] did an experiment in which he ingeniously hired subjects to participate who were purposefully misled. Each subject thought that his co-participants in each exercise were also subjects of the experimenter when in fact they were shills for him. The unsuspecting subjects participated in a group whose task was ostensibly to judge the relative lengths of lines drawn on a piece of paper.

The task was obvious and unsubtle; the lines differed from each other by .25 inch to 1.25 inches. Seven to nine men gave their opinion about which line was longer, with the naive subjects listening to the opinions of all of the others before their turn came up. The shills were told to give the same wrong answer unanimously. The subjects would have to be in direct opposition to the others if they decided to give the right answer.

In Asch's first experiment, an astonishing 37 percent of subjects gave the answer that conformed to the majority opinion. Most of the rest questioned their own judgment, not that of the others. Presumably the opinions of strangers were not of major consequence to these subjects, since they would have no further contact with them. If it were possible to design a similar experiment using important family members instead of strangers, I would predict with confidence that the number of subjects parroting the obviously wrong answer would be much higher than 37 percent.

In a study published in 1963, Stanley Milgram studied the willingness of otherwise moral and kind people to inflict pain on another person under the direction of an authority figure even though it ran against their normal pro-social impulses.[14] He set up an experiment in which a man would supposedly be punished for answering questions incorrectly by having subjects administer what appeared to be increasingly severe electric shocks. Milgram set up a machine that would appear to administer these shocks. He labeled the controls on the machine from "slight shock" to "danger: severe shock." In reality no shock was delivered at all, and the man who was being punished was an actor who communicated more and more severe distress as the experiment proceeded.

When subjects became uncomfortable and questioned the experimenter, the experimenter would prod them to continue using language that ranged from "please continue" to "you have no other choice, you *must* go on." Despite obvious discomfort, about 65 percent of the subjects obeyed the experimenter and went on to deliver the most severe shocks despite the screams from the actor.

One last well-known study in social psychology was conducted by Philip Zimbardo in 1971 and was called the *Stanford Prisoner Experiment*. The study was never published and the design has been criticized, especially because the experimenter may have unduly influenced the behavior of the subjects, but the results were nonetheless impressive and shocking. Twenty-four normal undergraduates were recruited to play the role of prisoners and guards for two weeks in a mock prison in the basement of a building. The experiment was halted after only six days. The subjects adapted to their roles so completely that one-third of the boys designated as guards began to become sadistic with the boys designated as prisoners. None of the guards had a previous history of antisocial behavior. Many of the prisoners accepted their fate after failed attempts at group rebellion, and some of them began to show severe emotional disturbances.

THE TIES THAT BIND: KIN SELECTION

If people are basically selfish and our biological imperative is to survive in order to pass down our genes to future generations, how do we explain the willingness of so many people to die for their country or their clan in a war? Throughout history, hundreds of thousands of men have marched headlong and almost without flinching into enemy spears, arrows, gunfire, and bombs, all the while watching their friends and comrades killed or maimed right beside them.

Individuals who die in battle are glorified by most societies as heroes. Mothers who send their sons off to war are also honored. In the United States, women whose sons die in war are hailed as "Gold Star Mothers." When I was growing up in the 1950s, other boys would come up to me and ask me if I was willing to die for my country in a war. Saying no meant being socially ostracized. The idea that maybe one should not always be willing to do that was rarely entertained anywhere in the world on a wide scale until opposition developed to the Vietnam War in the United States in the mid-1960s.

How do we explain the willingness of so many people to die for their families when they believe their families are under threat? Almost any one of us is willing to take a bullet to protect at least someone to whom we are strongly attached. On the other hand, if we are strongly motivated for our progeny to survive, how do we explain mothers in China who kill their own baby daughters in response to China's one-child policy? How do we explain the so-called honor killings in the Middle East, where otherwise loving fathers or brothers murder their own daughters or sisters because of social infractions that we in the United States consider minor or not infractions at all?

In a similar vein, what selfish explanation can be evoked to explain the behavior of Serbs, Croats, and Albanians in Yugoslavia as that country broke apart starting in the 1990s? These ethnic groups had lived together in peace for the previous forty years. They had been close neighbors and good friends, socializing together and intermarrying. Not too many years after the dictator Tito died, they turned on each other, killed each other, and "ethnically cleansed" entire cities.

I once asked a Croatian psychiatrist what he thought was the reason for these historical developments. He replied that, unlike Americans, people in that part of the world had long memories. I knew that the Croats and Serbs had been on opposite sides during World War II and had committed atrocities against one another, so his answer seemed to make some sense, since those events had happened in some folks' living memory.

As I thought more about my question and his answer, however, I had the disturbing thought that maybe he was also alluding to memories of the Battle of Kosovo Polje in 1389. After all, the Serbians kept bringing that up when the Albanians in Kosovo tried to gain their independence. That is a long time to carry a grudge. Yugoslavs may have long memories, but what happened to their short-term memory? Had they forgotten about the advantages they all accrued when they were friends living in peace? Are old memories more powerful than common sense?

These seemingly odd behaviors, where large numbers of people sacrifice themselves for their social groups and are perfectly willing to kill other people, even some from their own family, despite their own best interests, is extremely common historically. They must come very naturally to us *Homo sapiens*. Are they in our genes? I have been making the case throughout this chapter that genes do not determine specific behaviors, but they do cause us to have certain tendencies. We can override these tendencies, especially since we have evolved the ability to anticipate negative consequences to our behavior and change it accordingly. Still, if a behavior is as common as wars have been, and people often ignore all reason as they march off to them, we all must have some sort of strong genetic tendency to explain it.

If Charles Darwin's theory of natural selection, the passing on of genes due to the survival of the fittest, is a valid explanation for the phenomenon of evolution, then these behaviors must have evolved because the genes that predispose human beings toward them are more likely to be passed down than genes that do not. But how is that possible? Surely if you sacrifice yourself, you are less likely to pass down your genes. Ditto if you kill your own daughter. And going to war because of old historical injustices after enjoying the benefits of peace certainly endangers one's chances to reproduce in the future. Surely the people involved could easily remember the good times.

Darwin actually addressed this issue. At first the characteristic of altruism, the willingness to sacrifice oneself for the seeming good of one's ethnic or kin group, seemed to him to be at odds with his theory of natural selection. He then realized that this paradox would disappear if he changed his focus from the individual with a good genetic adaptation to the group to which the individual belonged. A single individual with a genetic mutation that is highly desirable and adaptive may still die before reproducing. If a group such as a family, a herd, or a tribe has many individuals who share the adaptation, then the propagation of that gene becomes far more likely. The survival of a genetic adaptation is dependent on the size of the number of individuals who share the genes, not just on the presence or absence of the gene in a single individual. If the individual organism's sacrifice of itself or its offspring helps a whole group to survive, the genes that predispose it to this behavior are selected for over time.

For example, if an individual deer in a herd breaks a leg and demands the attention of its family, and its relatives and the rest of the herd lovingly wait around for it to heal, then they all become easy target for predators, and the whole group may not survive. If, on the other hand, the injured deer's genetic predisposition allows it to altruistically sacrifice itself by going off into the forest to die, and the herd's genetic propensity is to metaphorically wish it good luck and move on to safer areas of the forest, the whole group is more likely to survive. The kin group of all the animals containing these genes becomes more likely to reproduce and pass on their altruistic genes to future generations. Under some circumstances, killing off one's own progeny will lead to enhanced survival for the group as a whole, so genes that predispose toward that behavior under some environmental contingencies would also be selected for through the forces of evolution.

In biology, this idea is known as *kin selection*. It remains controversial among evolutionary biologists and is not widely accepted by them, but I believe that its lack of acceptance has less to do with science and more to do with some of the same cultural forces that led to the predominance of psychoanalytic thinking over biological psychiatry in this country after World War II. Many biologists fear that the idea of kin selection could be misused in the way that the Nazis misused eugenics: to justify the killing off of weaker members of society or committing genocide against other ethnic groups who are viewed as genetically inferior. It could also be seen as a rationale for social Darwinism.

The idea that we may be willing to sacrifice our own interests for the good of our kin group is particularly difficult for Americans to accept. Because of the relative emphasis on individualism versus collectivism that has for so long been a defining characteristic of American culture, many of us find this idea almost ludicrous. We tend to believe that people are motivated entirely by selfishness. Even if people appear to be altruistic, we tend to think that they have some ulterior motive. Maybe they engage in selfless activities because it will gain praise for them, or will get them into heaven. Maybe even Mother Teresa did what she did entirely for the glory.

For centuries, societies have punished people who break the rules by exiling them from their communities. Today, families still disown wayward children in a way that parallels political exile. For many people, being thrown out of their kin or ethnic group or country is one of the most horrible punishments imaginable. It is literally a fate worse than death. Despite our fear, we can still choose to accept that fate rather than give in to the demands of our social network, but few of us are willing to make that choice.

If people are exiled or disowned, they often feel terribly alone and confused about who they really are. They begin to doubt their own choices, desires, and even their perceptions. They may become depressed or suicidal. I knew of a woman from India who defied her parents' desire for her to have an arranged marriage by planning to marry the American she fell in love with. She killed herself before she could follow through with her plan.

Tribalism

The forces of kin selection operate on human groups at both the large and the small group level. At the level of the ethnic group, people are willing to sacrifice themselves and even their families to protect the interests of the group. The best term for this tendency is *tribalism*. The term is not used much today, however, because it was differentially applied to nonwhite groups such as the ethnic groups of sub-Saharan Africa and not to European ethnic groups. Therefore, it took on the pejorative connotation that African peoples were more "primitive" than Europeans, and for that reason it became politically incorrect. It should rightly be applied as much to Serbs and Croats as to the Luo and Kikuyu of Kenya.

Because of the reluctance of the media to use the term, people in the United States developed some wrong-headed ideas about the fighting in African civil wars over the last fifty years. For example, during the Angolan Civil War between 1975 and 2002, the sides of the conflict were identified in the Western press by the superpower benefactors of the various factions. The Americans and the Soviets were in fact using different tribes to fight a proxy war. Thus, newspapers spoke of the FNLA and UNITA factions as "anticommunist" because they were supported by the United States. They were fighting the MPLA, which was identified as a "communist" group because it was backed by the Soviets. Actually, the political philosophies of the groups were not all that different. MPLA fighters mostly belonged to the Kimbundu tribe, FNLA fighters to the Bakonga family of tribes, and UNITA fighters to the Ovimbundu family of tribes.

The history of using tribalism to advance the interests of outside powers dates all the way back to the Treaty of Berlin in 1884. The European colonial powers divided the African continent into "countries" that purposely disregarded tribal boundaries. Often tribes that were centuries-old enemies were combined in the same country. The colonial power would then further inflame tribal conflict by favoring the members of one tribe over another under a strategy known as "divide and rule." The fact that a historical event from so long ago continues to create chaos today is testament to the power of kin selection.

Self-Sacrifice

At the level of the family, the forces of kin selection are expressed by the tendency of individuals to give up their own idiosyncratic desires in order to play a specific role within their families that seems to advance the needs of the group. If necessary, individuals are even willing to die or to kill other family members if the viability of the family is under threat and the sacrifice seems to be necessary for the family to survive or prosper.

In my writings, I have made the case that people who are self-destructive cannot be acting out of selfish motives. That is literally a contradiction in terms, and sounds to me like doublethink straight out of the novel *1984*. Still, most schools of psychological thought try to find a selfish motive for those who act in a self-defeating manner. Maybe these people *enjoy* pain. They could be masochists. Pain is pleasure? The rest of us tend to attribute such behavior to the person's insanity, wickedness, or downright stupidity. As we shall see later in the chapter on psychotherapy, a few theorists have proposed that people are sometimes motivated to behave in ways that are contrary to their own interests or happiness because they believe that this behavior is necessary to preserve their families in some way.

Black Sheep

If these ideas about kin selection are true, some readers may protest, then what about those individuals who revel in being black sheep? Many people go out of their way to defy their families. They do the opposite of what they are told. Mental health professionals use the term "oppositional" to describe them. Children are even said to have "oppositional defiant disorder." Maybe it is a mental illness. I do not think so. I think oppositional families members act that way because *that is what they think their families expect of them.* They are going along with the program every bit as much as those family members who do exactly what they are told. They do not make their own independent choices; they feel they *must* do the opposite of what they are told.

The neglect of family dynamics since the family systems therapists started to lose their prominent position in psychotherapy circles after the 1980s not only helped usher in the era of biological psychiatry but also set back psychotherapy. Disregard of social influences on the psyche had been a major weakness of most schools of thought in psychotherapy even before systems ideas, and it still is. This will be the subject of Chapter Nine. In the next chapter, I will discuss how a movement extolling the virtues of so-called "evidence-based medicine" in psychiatry and psychology has entered the mix of factors leading to the devaluation of social behavior as a major factor in contributing to many psychological and social problems.

6

Evidence-Based Ignorance

The social and economic factors that pushed the mental health field away from a treatment focus on family and other interpersonal relationship problems and toward Band-Aid approaches such as purely symptom-oriented treatments got yet another boost with demands from the public, managed care insurance companies, and academic psychology departments for so-called *evidence-based* treatment interventions.

MEDICAL ERRORS

Starting in early 1999, statistics about patient deaths from preventable medical errors started to become widely known and began to raise alarm bells in both the public and in the medical establishment. The Institute of Medicine (IOM) issued a report in 2000[1] called *To Err Is Human* estimating that such errors caused between 44,000 and 98,000 fatalities per year. These numbers are higher than the number of yearly deaths from automobile accidents or breast cancer. Many of these fatal medical errors occur in hospitals, particularly during surgery. The patient receives the wrong anesthesia or a surgical sponge is left in the patient after he or she has been sewn up. A significant number of medical errors also take place in doctors' offices.

The immediate culprit in the minds of the medical establishment was an allegedly inadequate system of medical education. Medical educators were not, according to this line of thought, keeping up with new developments in the field and with changing medical systems of care such as electronic medical records and briefer hospital stays.

The national body that accredits residency training programs in all specialties, the Accreditation Council for Graduate Medical Education (ACGME), jumped into action extremely quickly, even before the final report of the IOM, to address this issue. The ACGME "core competencies" project was approved at the end of September 1999, and implementation of its first phase was to be completed by 2001.

The project designates six areas of specific knowledge, skills, and attitudes, and the ACGME mandates that all six are to be taught explicitly in all residency programs. Trainees are also supposed to be "reliably" evaluated on their performance in these six areas, appropriate to their individual specialties, despite the fact that no reliable methods for evaluating these competencies have ever been published that are any better than observation by faculty members of a resident's clinical performance. That was of course already being done. The six general competencies are patient care, medical knowledge, self-improvement based on practice and continuing education, interpersonal and communication skills, professionalism, and the understanding of modern medical systems of care.

I cannot speak for other directors of residency programs, but my experience was that medical education did not improve a whole lot in response to these new mandates. What changed was the amount of paperwork that was required of faculty members. They created several new evaluation forms for each resident that I had to nag faculty members to turn in. This paperwork takes time away from teaching. More important, the emphasis of the ACGME on training as a response to medical errors ignores what I believe to be a much more important reason for physician mistakes.

As I have already discussed, the increasing financial pressures on doctors from managed care insurance companies have led doctors to spend less and less time with each patient they treat. This has resulted in a lack of time for clinicians to properly evaluate a patient. In psychiatry, this in turn has led to the employment of various diagnostic shortcuts that shortchange the evaluation of psychosocial factors that might lead to different diagnostic considerations. The patient's current family environment is given precious little attention. Some of the shortcuts employed by psychiatrists and their effects will be discussed in Chapter Seven.

While the use of these shortcuts may still lead to adequate care in routine cases, in more complicated cases they can lead to disastrous misdiagnoses and the inappropriate use of potentially dangerous medications. Furthermore, the lack of time and the need to see more patients lead to physician fatigue, which also increases the odds that a doctor will make a serious error of judgment. On top of that, doctors are facing more and more paperwork, which either increases their overhead expenses for office help or takes away even more time from treating patients.

Government and insurance companies continue to lead the charge for physician "improvement." In their efforts to reassure the public that they are taking the problem of bad doctors seriously, they have begun to institute a grading system for individual practitioners that is to be made available to the public. Doctors will be asked to turn in evidence that they ordered certain tests or provided certain treatments that should be the standard of practice for the treatment of particular illnesses. Insurance companies will also use incentive pay for those doctors (*performance-based pay*) who appear to be conscientious and competent in doing what should be required of them based on these reports. Eventually, report cards on a doctor's record of treatment outcomes for specific disorders may be added to the mix.

This process sounds like a good thing for the public, but once again it will create financial pressures on doctors that will take time away from patient care, cause them to hire more clerical help, which raises costs, or see more patients to make up for the financial hit they will take. They may do all or any combination of these things. My prediction is that performance-based pay will increase rather than decrease the number of preventable medical errors. Furthermore, if report cards on doctors' outcomes with their patients are issued, this will discourage doctors from treating difficult or complex cases. Good results are more likely to occur in patients with uncomplicated disorders, so a strong financial incentive will be present for doctors to treat only those patients and send away the tough cases.

WHAT CONSTITUTES EVIDENCE?

In the field at large, the latest trend in medicine in general and psychiatry in particular is for regulatory bodies and insurance companies to insist that doctors must solely employ something called *evidence-based medicine*. The use of this term implies that much of what some doctors do, particularly psychiatrists and psychologists, is not based on scientific evidence but something else entirely, and that these other practices must be stopped.

Usually "evidence" as used in this way is meant to consist entirely of what is considered the highest standard of evidence in medical science: the *randomized, double-blind, placebo-controlled* study using a large and *homogeneous* (nearly identical in many important ways) sample of patients. I will define these terms shortly for readers who are unfamiliar with them. One single such study is considered only tentative evidence for the efficacy of a treatment. In order to become accepted fact, such studies require *replication*, or the finding of similar results in several similar experiments.

The something that is supposedly not evidence-based is termed *anecdotal* evidence, or evidence based on an individual practitioner's clinical experiences with individual cases. This sort of evidence is just assumed to be biased by the preconceived notions of the doctor or perhaps based on atypical patients. According to this line of reasoning, anecdotal evidence is therefore unreliable if not completely worthless. Somehow years of clinical experience with successes and failures of different treatment modalities in a variety of different patients in different populations and contexts have been completely discounted in some medical circles.

The editors of a few journals do recognize that clinical anecdotes may have some validity. They publish *case reports,* which describe a clinician's experience with a single case. Usually only the most unusual cases are published—stories about patients with rare symptoms, often jokingly referred to by medical educators as "zebras." Occasionally a case report is published because it seems to bring the conventional wisdom about some clinical disorder into question. Many journals do not publish case reports or relegate them to the rarely read letters to the editor section of the journal.

Evidence for the Efficacy of Psychotherapy

Virtually this same argument about the validity of clinical experience versus "experimental" evidence broke out among psychotherapists in the American Psychological Association years before the medical errors scare pushed its way into the consciousness of psychiatrists. Starting in 1993, leaders of Division 12 of the organization, called the Society of Clinical Psychology, pushed the notion that "acceptable" research should be limited to include only randomized clinical trials or, occasionally, single-subject study designs under highly controlled conditions. Clinical reports were again said to be biased and unscientific.

Behind the demands for "evidence" was a surreptitious attack on more humanistically based treatment in favor of a type of psychotherapy called cognitive-behavior therapy or CBT, which has gained ascendancy in most psychology training programs. This form of therapy has a larger number of studies demonstrating efficacy than any other psychotherapy model. I believe this is because, in its original form, CBT is relatively straightforward, oriented toward symptoms rather than persons, and far easier to study than therapies that deal with complex human relationships and subtle mental processes. Even so, CBT studies have significant methodological problems, and often show statistically rather than clinically significant results. This does not mean that such studies should not be done or should be disregarded, but rather that they are but one of many valid forms of scientific observation.

Much of human behavior, relationships, psychological processes, and psychotherapy methodology is simply not amenable to traditional scientific study designs. First, we cannot read minds, so scientists have to infer what is going on in there from the patient's overt behavior or from what patients say about themselves. The psychological effects of interpersonal and family relationships in particular are virtually impossible to study strictly within the parameters of most *empirical* or supposedly unbiased scientific studies. This is because of their staggering complexity.

For example, how is it possible to precisely measure and quantify how individuals in a relationship understand and react to the shades of meanings involved in their verbal and nonverbal communication? It cannot be done. During any relationship, the feelings, thoughts, and intensions of each individual, as well as their ideas about the feelings, thoughts, and intensions of the other person, are constantly in flux as ongoing feedback from the interpersonal environment is perceived and processed. Additionally, memories of events from the entire history of any relationship are figured in to the assessment of relationship events by the principals. This prior history continually affects each person's ideas about what is transpiring in the present and how he or she should respond to it. Two people in a relationship are engaged in an ongoing, complex, unscripted, and intricate dance in which they may be attempting to outmaneuver one another.

While every encounter between the two people in the relationship has familiar elements, every encounter is also somewhat different, and therefore different and at times novel responses are required. The understanding of these continual feedback loops between two persons in a relationship is one of the strengths of family systems theories and therapy, as will be described in Chapter Nine. The multiplicity of forms that results in both the uniqueness of each encounter *and* the repetitiveness of themes within encounters can be best appreciated in the context of an ongoing relationship between an observer and the observed.

Family members will often not even tell therapists or researchers the truth about what is transpiring within their family until they develop a trusting relationship with them. Developing trust can take weeks or months. If people see a researcher for a relatively brief interview, this will never happen. Even after trust has developed, much information is at first omitted. Trained therapists can pick up on recurring tendencies and problematic behavior only by listening to the stories patients tell about themselves.

Pattern Recognition

Humanistically oriented therapists listen to countless little stories patients tell about their relationships. When patients are asked to *free-associate* about their psychological problems—that is, report their thoughts in stream-of-consciousness form without self-censorship—they recount an average of three little relationship vignettes per hour.[2] As the therapist hears more and more of these stories, subtle repetitive patterns begin to become apparent. The longer patients stay in therapy, the better the therapist is able to understand them and the nature of these recurring patterns in their lives.

This sort of pattern recognition is something computers are not able to do well, at least so far, because recognizing them requires an understanding of common themes that recur in stories that may superficially sound unrelated. Such patterns are also unlikely to emerge in a single diagnostic interview or a psychological test of any sort. Engaging in long-term psychotherapy with a patient is not only the best way to elicit recurring patterns, but in many cases may be the only way.

Repetitive relationship patterns are understood by looking for what are termed *core conflictual relationship themes*.[2] Transcripts of audiotaped psychotherapy sessions can actually be reliably scored for the appearance of such themes—by people, not by computers. A session is scored by looking at three variables within the relationship vignettes that the patient provides: descriptions of wishes for certain outcomes within relationships, descriptions of the patient's own actual behavior toward others, and descriptions of how others generally respond to the patient.

Themes involve such things as dominance versus submission or wishes for closeness versus wishes for more distance. The scoring involves both how many times certain themes recur and whether the themes conflict with one another in some way. Wishes, for example, can conflict with what actually takes place in relationships in the other two spheres, or they can conflict with each other. This is one way to reliably measure ambivalence and intrapsychic conflict. Doing so requires multiple observations within an ongoing psycho-therapy relationship with a patient. The nature of the conflict will usually not emerge in a single encounter.

Any Research Method Can Be Used Well or Be Used Poorly

Even when psychological therapies per se are amenable to sup-posedly empirical studies, not all studies are created equal. Neither are all clinical anecdotes. Both anecdotal evidence *and* empirical studies can be easily and dramatically biased and manipulated. Anecdotal evidence can be relatively unbiased as well as very impor-tant. One can argue that the plural of *anecdote* is in many instances *empirical data.*

In the context of experimental studies in mental health, much of the data on subjects are really nothing more than a collection of anecdotes. For instance, how a subject responds to a psychological test at a given sitting is very similar to how a given patient responds to an intervention at a particular time in a psychotherapy session. An important factor, but not the only one, in determining the valid-ity of any data is how often the same observation repeats itself over an extended period of time in a reasonable number of similar subjects.

Another point to keep in mind is that the very first step in the scientific method is observation. Before one can design an experi-ment, one has to observe patterns that suggest on what it might be useful to experiment, and under what conditions the experiment should be done.

The validity of some anecdotes was illustrated by a tongue-in-cheek journal article[3] by G. C. Smith and J. P. Pell circulating on the Internet, entitled "Parachute Use to Prevent Death and Major Trauma Related to Gravitational Challenge: Systematic Review of [Randomized] Controlled Trials." The authors pointed out, after a review of the literature, that there are no randomized placebo-controlled studies that prove that parachutes prevent deaths or injuries for people who fall out of airplanes. A placebo is an inter-vention known to be ineffective.

They concluded: "As with many interventions intended to prevent ill health, the effectiveness of parachutes has not been subjected to rig-orous evaluation by using randomized controlled trials. Advocates of evidence-based medicine have criticized the adoption of interventions evaluated by using only observational data. We think that every-one might benefit if the most radical protagonists of evidence-based medicine organized and participated in a double blind, randomized, placebo controlled, crossover trial of the parachute."

This chapter will look at sources of bias in recent psychiatric and psychological discourse and publications, as well as describe under what circumstances anecdotes can provide useful scientific information. Before doing this, however, I will briefly define for those readers who are unfamiliar with them the design characteristics that are considered to be essential in empirical clinical studies. Any of these characteristics can be manipulated by an experimenter to stack the deck in favor of one result or another, often in very subtle ways. If the necessary elements of clinical trials are already part of your working knowledge, please feel free to skip this section and go on to the section called "Sources of Bias in Drug Studies."

"Empirical" Studies

The best type of clinical study compares an as yet unproven treatment for patients who manifest a particular psychiatric disorder with either a placebo or another treatment that is already known to be effective. In drug studies, the placebo is often a sugar pill, and it is made to look exactly like the experimental pill. The first step in a study is to employ reliable techniques to make sure that subjects actually have the psychiatric diagnosis or trait under study. These subjects are then divided into two groups. One group receives the experimental treatment and the other group receives either a placebo or the active treatment.

A study comparing a new treatment to one that is already known to be effective can of course only be done if an effective treatment already exists. If it does, this type of study is much better than a placebo study because it answers two questions instead of one: Is the experimental treatment effective, and is it *better* than the existing treatment? "Better" can mean more effective, but it can also mean that the new treatment has fewer side effects. For reasons that will become apparent shortly, most new drugs released on the market are *not* compared to other active drugs but to placebos.

The group receiving the placebo or the alternate treatment is called the *control group*. The *sample size* is the total number of subjects in the experiment, and also the numbers assigned to each of the two groups. The two groups should be very similar in all important ways so that the experimenter is not comparing apples to oranges.

Homogeneity of the sample is established in three ways. First, studies have *inclusion* and *exclusion* criteria that filter out potential subjects who may have characteristics that could cause the results of the study to be skewed. Second, the groups are compared in terms of things like demographics (age, race, gender, and so forth), earlier treatments, and the seriousness of the disorder being studied to see if the groups are comparable. Third, a statistical technique called *randomization* is used to make certain that assignment to a particular treatment is completely a matter of chance rather than the choice of a potentially biased experimenter.

Double blind means that neither the person who provides the treatment in the experiment nor the patients receiving the treatment know whether they are receiving the experimental treatment or the alternative. The person running the experiment should therefore not be the same person as the one who is providing the treatment. This technique is meant to cancel out the *placebo effect*. Patients' expectations about whether or not a drug will work, as well as whether or not the drug will have harmful side effects, are very important factors in determining whether patients will feel better, worse, or the same.

In most cases, there is no way to know how vulnerable any given patient is to having his or her results based more on his or her expectations than on the actual effectiveness of the experimental treatment. If the sample size is sufficiently large and randomization is done well, researchers assume that expectation effects will be about equal in the two groups and will cancel one another out in the statistical analysis of the results. However, this is not always the case. Since most drugs have significant side effects, subjects who get no side effects from a pill can easily figure out that they are getting the placebo.

Last, *outcome measures* are the supposedly "objective" measures of change in the psychological variables that are believed to be helped by the intervention or interventions under study. These measures can consist of observations made by the experimenter, changes in the results of laboratory tests, or changes in answers to *self-report* psychological tests. In the latter, the patients rate themselves on a variety of dimensions, such as the presence and severity of various symptoms, or their ability to function at work.

SOURCES OF BIAS IN DRUG STUDIES

When I was a young man, I admired and idealized scientists. Here was one field of human endeavor, I believed, where practitioners used actual evidence and rigorous methodologies before making claims about what has been proven to be true and what is mythology. Although I knew in the back of my head that scientists are human just like everyone else, I tended to continue to idealize scientists as I progressed through medical school, began my practice, and then became an academic psychiatrist myself. It was only later that I was confronted by impossible-to-deny evidence that scientists frequently manipulate their results for a number of ulterior purposes.

They may want to justify a preexisting point of view. They clearly play political games in academic centers and medical schools—known collectively as *academic politics*—to one-up one another or to further their own careers at the expense of others. In positions of power, some scientists routinely block either the funding for studies or the publication of data that is not in line with their prejudices or professional reputation.

A story in *The New Yorker* dated July 23, 2001,[4] was particularly eye opening. It reported that just one scientist literally blocked progress in the field of neuroscience for quite a few years. This one powerful man believed, as most people were then taught, that birds and mammals are born with all the brain cells they will ever have and that new neuron generation or regeneration never takes place in adults. He systematically blocked the publication of data that suggested that new production of neurons was in fact taking place. The careers of some scientists who tried to show this were stalled; others became so frustrated that they just decided to quit the field altogether. Finally, as the evidence gradually became so massive it could not be ignored, the guru had to back down. The generation of new neurons, under some circumstances and in some brain regions, does indeed occur even in the adult human brain.

Collusion between Academics and Big Pharma

Besides being motivated by power and prestige, scientists also bias their results because many of them, just like the rest of us in other walks of life, are greedy. In particular, researchers can sometimes be literally bribed into producing research results that are consistent with the plans of the marketing divisions of very well-funded pharmaceutical companies. Usually, when evidence of such bias is discovered, researchers who seem to do this are given the benefit of the doubt by the field at large. They are thought to have been suckered in by the drug company and to be "in denial" that they are doing anything purely for financial gain. I tend to be more cynical, and think that many of them are doing the bidding of big pharma quite willingly. For example, many researchers will allow the drug companies to control the design of their clinical trials without protest, even when design flaws are obvious.[5]

I have already mentioned some drug company marketing tactics earlier in this volume. Here I will focus mostly on the collusion of the scientists who are involved in biasing the perceptions of mental health clinicians about what constitutes "evidenced-based" practice. While the fact that researchers have a conflict of interest does not in itself prove that the results of a given study are biased, it does make its results suspect. Later on, when I discuss the current horrific trend of diagnosing very young children with bipolar disorder and treating them with very powerful and toxic medications, I will mention a particularly startling example.

If anyone questions whether pharmaceutical companies bias the results of their clinical trials, some basic facts should make it exceeding clear. At least three published surveys have looked at how company-sponsored clinical trials turn out. Most such trials only compare a new drug to a placebo, because that is all the FDA requires for them to approve the drug. The company just has to show that a drug works, not that it is better or worse than any existing treatment. For placebo-controlled studies in psychiatry, one survey[6] showed that almost half had at least one author who was in the drug manufacturer's direct employ. The studies in which such was the case were five times as likely to report a positive result as studies in which it was not.

In the few situations where two active drugs are compared to one another for efficacy, another survey[7] reported that 89 to 98 percent found results favorable to the sponsor's product rather than a competitor's similar product. Yet another similar study[8] found that 90 percent of studies comparing two of the new antipsychotic medications came out in favor of the sponsor's drug. These percentages are far too high to be due entirely to chance. Any doubts about this last statement should be erased by the last study mentioned. In this survey of the literature, drug A was found to be superior to drug B in some studies, while drug B was found to be superior to drug C in others. Drug C in yet other studies was found to be superior to drug A! At drug company–sponsored dinner talks, only the studies favorable to the manufacturer's drug are generally mentioned.

Any study design variable can be manipulated in ways that can almost guarantee a final result that is in line with whatever biases the chief experimenter would like to see. The way diagnoses are made, the way groups are compared, and the way results are measured can lead to highly misleading conclusions. I will be mentioning examples of the way study designers have bent study results in their favor later in this chapter and the chapters that follow. Right now, I will focus on how the publication of data can be manipulated and distributed in ways highly likely to mislead clinicians, resulting in their prescribing widely accepted but nonetheless spurious, dangerous, or unnecessary treatments for patients when better alternatives are available.

MISLEADING ABSTRACTS AND OVERSTATEMENT OF THE RESULTS OF STUDIES

Through the misuse of the way an article in a scientific journal is structured, doctors can be misled on a large scale. This presence of this tactic also provides good evidence that researchers may be actively complicit with drug company marketing needs or are purposely misleading practicing clinicians in order to build their careers.

Clinicians, tending to be busy sorts, do not have a lot of time to read journals. Authors and publishers of journals know this. To "help" doctors with this problem, writers of journal articles thoughtfully insert at the beginning of each article an abstract or summary of the methods, findings, and conclusions contained in the body of the article. Articles also end with a discussion of what the data presented by the authors might signify. The discussion section of the paper routinely includes any potential weaknesses in the study's design or subject selection that may have biased the results. However, it is rare that all of the study weaknesses discussed in this section of the paper are mentioned in the abstract, so that clinicians who only read the abstract are not aware of factors that might bring the study's conclusions into question.

Not infrequently, the conclusions presented in the abstract of a journal article do not accurately reflect the data presented in the body of the article. Sometimes, the conclusions in the abstract are not even supported by the data at all.

Within the discussion section in the body of the article, significant potential weaknesses of the study are at times not mentioned at all. They can be ascertained only through an extremely careful reading of the paper. To further complicate matters, when the study's conclusions are presented at professional meetings, informally discussed by clinicians, or discussed in articles in psychiatric newspapers and certain publications, the strength of the conclusions may be grossly exaggerated, and tentative conclusions presented as undisputed facts.

I will now discuss an illustrative example. This example is indirectly related to the issue of the neglect of psychosocial variables in much of today's psychiatry, as I will explain after showing how the paper and its abstract are misleading. The article clearly demonstrates the tactics I have just mentioned. The article is called "Effectiveness of Adjunctive Antidepressant Treatment for Bipolar Depression," and it was published in the *New England Journal of Medicine* on April 26, 2007.[9] The article has been *cited* (quoted) extensively. To help the reader fully appreciate how this misleading article became so influential, I must first discuss the relative prestige of various medical journals and what that means to the average clinician, as well as some relevant characteristics of the diagnosis of bipolar depression. If these phenomena are already well known to you, you are encouraged to skip the next two sections and go directly to the section entitled "Issues in the Treatment of Bipolar Depression."

Prestige Journals

All scientific and medical journals are not created equal in the minds of doctors in terms of their prestige and the seriousness with which results published in the journal are taken. In fact, some journals are known as "throwaway journals" because they are of relatively low value. Such journals are usually mailed free of charge, and some of them are fully controlled by big pharma.

Almost all journals accept some drug company advertising to help manage production and distribution costs, and that fact may influence which studies get published and which do not, although the more prestigious journals contain limited ads or none at all. The better journals are *peer-reviewed*, meaning that articles submitted to the journal for publication are reviewed and screened by several experts in the field for content and scientific validity before they are accepted. Peer reviewers can recommend changes in the article that need to be made prior to publication, or they can recommend rejection of a study for publication altogether.

Various peer-reviewed journals are ranked in the minds of practitioners by how prestigious they are believed to be. The most prestigious journals are thought to have the very highest standards. They are taken the most seriously by the majority of doctors. Because of their reputation, the high-prestige journals reject a higher percentage of submissions and are therefore more difficult for scientists to get their studies published in. The *New England Journal of Medicine* is near the top of the food chain for all of medicine, not just for psychiatry. Therefore, the example I will describe is particularly bothersome.

Bipolar Depression

Let me now briefly discuss the diagnosis of bipolar depression. I will discuss the other forms of depression later, since diagnosis figures prominently in misleading debates over whether pharmacology, psychotherapy, or some combination is the best treatment for depression. An episode of the most serious syndrome of depression is known as a *major depressive episode* and is characterized by a certain level of severity and pervasiveness as well as by the number of symptoms of depression that are present.

Major depressive episodes that are not caused directly by a reaction to a drug or by a medical illness that affects the brain come in two varieties: unipolar and bipolar. Unipolar depressions are those in which the patient's mood only swings downward from normal into depression. Bipolar depressions, on the other hand, are part of bipolar disorder or manic-depressive illness. The afflicted individuals have both major depressive episodes, or lows, and severe highs (*manic episodes*). Both major depressive episodes and manic episodes are usually self-limited, which means that they eventually go away without treatment. They usually recur sometime later. In other words, patients with these disorders have significantly long periods during which they have a normal range of moods. I will again discuss the diagnosis of bipolar disorder later on in the volume, as the diagnosis—or more correctly the misdiagnosis—of the disorder has become a fad in the field of psychiatry.

Issues in the Treatment of Bipolar Depression

Unipolar depression is treated with a variety of antidepressant drugs. All of these medications are approximately of equal effectiveness in the sense that the percentage of patients responding well to the different ones is approximately the same (their manufacturers may argue otherwise), although a given patient may respond to some of them but not to others. In individual studies, antidepressants do not seem to be much more effective than placebo, but those studies are misleading, as I will soon demonstrate.

The antidepressants have also been used since the 1950s to treat bipolar depression. Most clinicians I know have used them successfully for years. In my experience, they are often at least if not more effective in bipolar depression than they are in unipolar depression. This is because bipolar depressive episodes tend to exhibit characteristics of a subtype of major depression known as melancholia more frequently than do unipolar depressive episodes. The more symptoms of melancholia that are present in a given case, in my own clinical experience and in that of every other clinician I know, the more likely the depression is to respond to antidepressant medication. Melancholic depression is also far less likely to respond to placebo than other varieties, and it does not respond at all to psychotherapy.

When patients who are known to have bipolar disorder are placed on an antidepressant all by itself, they may very quickly "switch" into a high or manic episode. This can be quite dangerous, as patients in a manic state can destroy their lives through extreme and thoughtless impulsivity. However, if these patients are first put on a "mood stabilizer" drug (lithium, Depakote, Tegretol, or any antipsychotic medication) to which they are known responders, they do not switch. This observation was actually one of the conclusions of the study I am about to criticize. That conclusion was well supported by the data in the study. Another one of the study's conclusions was not so well supported.

In recent years, articles have been printed and lectures given that maintain that the use of antidepressants in bipolar disorder should be contraindicated, meaning that it should be a no-no. This seems to be part of a widespread campaign, mentioned in Chapter Four, to generally discredit antidepressants initiated after most of the newest ones went off patent. In bipolar disorder, the problem that they may cause switching into mania is often advanced as one justification for this "contraindication," usually by writers who forget to mention that mood stabilizers can prevent switching from taking place. The drugs are also accused of inducing *rapid cycling* or even *ultra rapid cycling*, meaning that they supposedly cause bipolar patients to suddenly start to quickly and chronically cycle between depressive and manic episodes, with no breaks in between. Ultra rapid cycling is said to be almost impossible to treat.

Now, in over thirty years of clinical experience with inpatients and outpatients, and in the experience of all the residents I have directly supervised over the years, I have never seen that happen. Perhaps it is extremely rare and I just have not come across a case. I have never seen a case of a serious but rare side effect of antipsychotic medication called neuromalignant syndrome (NMS), but I do believe it exists. The people who talk about ultra rapid cycling, however, claim it is anything but rare, but hey, maybe I have just been lucky.

Coincidently, the warning about the dangers of antidepressants in bipolar disorder reached a crescendo around the time that most of them became available in cheaper but equally effective generic forms rather than solely as expensive brand-name drugs. Meanwhile, clinical trials have begun to show that the newer antipsychotic drugs may be somewhat effective in treating bipolar depression. Most of these drugs are still only available as the expensive brand-name versions; the older antipsychotics that are off patent have of course never been tested for this indication.

Big pharma makes big profits if expensive brand-name drugs are used in place of cheap generic alternatives. Could this be behind the recent criticism of the use of antidepressants in bipolar depression? I do not know for certain; I will let the reader be the judge.

A more recent and even more surprising criticism of the use of antidepressants in bipolar depression is that they are just plain ineffective. Two or three journal articles have purported to show this. I found this conclusion quite perplexing in light of my clinical experience and the fact that other studies have been published that show that the drugs do work. However, one of the contrary articles appeared in the highly prestigious *New England Journal* mentioned above, so I thought I might have to reconsider my view.

This article concluded that antidepressants were no better than placebo in bipolar depression. Placebo helped 27.3 percent of subjects, while the antidepressants helped only 23.5 percent. I suspected something might be wrong with the study design, even though these data at first sounded very impressive to me. Then I carefully read the actual article.

In the study described by the article, the deck seemed to have indeed been stacked in favor of the study turning out the way it did. This slight-of-hand was accomplished through the way that subjects for the study were selected. Although this potentially serious bias could be ascertained by reading between the lines in the section of the article that describes the study's methods, no direct mention of it is made in either the abstract or in the section of the paper that described the study's weaknesses. The conclusions of the study, if adopted by large numbers of psychiatrists, would lead to the increased use of brand-name medications that are less effective, have much worse side effects, and are more expensive than generic antidepressants.

The Misleading Abstract

In this study, subjects with bipolar depression did not respond well to either one of two different antidepressant medications when they were added to preexisting therapy with mood-stabilizing drugs. I first looked to see if all of the medications used by the study subjects—both the antidepressants and the mood stabilizers—were given at an adequate dosage and for an adequate duration. If they had not been, then the study results would have been questionable.

Underdosing a competitor's drug or using it for an inadequate period of time is a frequent tactic used in clinical trials sponsored by pharmaceutical companies to tout the superiority of their drug over a competitor's "me-too" drug. However, everything looked just dandy in this regard.

I again started to question my sanity. I did notice near the end of the article, on page 1,720, that the authors pointed out that some of the study subjects had been previously receiving clinical treatment at "participating sites." I then went back and reread the article more carefully. This time, on the bottom of page 1,713, I noticed a couple of curious things.

First, it said that "standard" antidepressants that were already in use by subjects prior to inclusion in the study were tapered off over a two-week period. This means that some of the subjects were already taking other antidepressants besides the two used in the study, of which quite a few are available, and were not responding to them. Second, only patients who had previously not responded to either of the two antidepressants used in the study were excluded from the study entirely. The number of subjects who had not responded to one of the many other antidepressants was not specified in the article. Since all of the study subjects were diagnosed as being in the midst of an active bipolar depressive episode at the start of the study, this meant that some of the study subjects had *already* been unresponsive to treatment with at least one antidepressant before the study had even started.

I searched the "selection of subjects" section of the article and the printed tables comparing the baseline characteristics of subjects in the groups being compared in vain to find out exactly what percentage of the subjects had thusly been unresponsive to previous treatment. In order to understand why this is significant, some other characteristics of antidepressant therapy first need to be understood.

One of the reasons that antidepressants are so useful clinically when studies seem to show that they are barely better than placebo is that, in studies, the drugs are not used the way clinicians use them. In the vast majority of drug studies, only one antidepressant is used. If it fails, as will any drug from any class given to patients with any medical disorder, nothing else is done. In practice, however, if one antidepressant does not work in a given patient after sufficient increases in dosages and duration of treatment, clinicians then switch the patient to a different one. Such patients often will respond to the second drug. We do not really know why certain patients respond to one agent over another, but every patient is different in this regard.

One large study known as the STAR*D[10] study attempted to study antidepressants in the way that clinicians actually use them. It found that indeed a second antidepressant can work if a first one fails. A third or fourth may work if the first two or three fail, and so forth. The total percentage of depressed patients who respond to antidepressant drugs is therefore the percentage of people who respond to the first drug plus the percentage of those who respond to the second and so forth. This total ends up being a very high percentage of the initial group.

However, the law of diminishing returns applies. The percentage of additional patients who respond to the next agent used falls quickly as initially unresponsive patients are moved from the first to the second to the third agent. In the STAR*D study, only 30.6 percent of patients who failed a trial of one drug responded to the second agent used.

If a large percentage of the patients in the *New England Journal* study on bipolar depression were already nonresponders to at least one antidepressant—and once again I was unable to ascertain what the actual numbers were since they were not published—then of course many would be found to be nonresponders to the antidepressants in the study! This is especially true since any single antidepressant studied alone tends to barely outdo placebo to begin with.

I e-mailed the main author of the study to see if he had the data on what percentage of subjects in his study had failed previous trials of antidepressants. So far I have not received a reply. The point I am making here is that it seems peculiar that this important information was not published in the article. Moreover, the poor responder status of at least some subjects was not mentioned in the section of the article dealing with the weaknesses of the study.

The second peculiarity mentioned on page 1,713 had to do with the use of the aforementioned antipsychotic medications, which may be helpful in ameliorating bipolar depression. They are already well known to be extremely effective in treating mania. In fact, they may be the most effective mood stabilizers around, because the drugs that are actually called mood stabilizers really are, in clinical experience, much better at preventing manic episodes in bipolar patients than they are at preventing depressive episodes.

The study in the *New England Journal* took place between November 1999 and July 2005. Prior to 2004, only users of the mood stabilizers lithium, Depakote, Tegretol, or some combination thereof were allowed in the study. After 2004, the protocol was changed to allow the use of any FDA-approved antimanic drugs. According to the Web site Medscape, around the beginning of that year, some of the new (so-called *atypical*) antipsychotics received the FDA indication for the treatment of mania. The old antipsychotics, always known clinically to work in mania, had never been studied for this indication, and therefore do not have the FDA's approval for this use. These "typicals" were all available as generics at the time that the drug companies received the FDA-blessed indication for mania for their atypicals.

Since we now think that atypicals may help bipolar depression, and since some of the study subjects were already taking them at the time of the initiation of the study, this meant that some percentage of the subjects might have been especially resistant to *any* treatment for bipolar depression.

Now I do not know if the authors of the study were aware in 2004 of any of the studies showing that the atypicals are useful for depression. The timing does seem curious. I do know that a colleague of mine used to use low doses of an old antipsychotic drug called Navane as an add-on treatment to antidepressants for unipolar or bipolar patients because he believed that it enhanced or *potentiated* their beneficial effects. That was way back in 1978.

All the authors of the *New England Journal* study had multiple financial ties to several pharmaceutical companies, many of which had recently lost patents on their antidepressants but still had active patents on their version of the atypicals. Again, this last fact does not prove that the authors were being dishonest, or if they were, that they were dishonest for this specific reason, but one must certainly wonder.

The Aftermath of the Misleading Abstract

The results of the studies that purportedly showed antidepressants to be ineffective in bipolar depression created a lot of talk between both clinicians and the "experts" in the field. As these discussions continued, many psychiatrists began to speak of its conclusion as if it were a well-established fact. For example, in response to a letter to the editor to the prestigious *American Journal of Psychiatry* in August of 2008[11] (even letters to the editors of high-prestige journals are subject to peer review), three physicians, using the *New England Journal* article as a reference, stated that "a major finding of [this study] was that antidepressants appear to have no benefit beyond that of mood stabilizers alone in the treatment of bipolar depression, despite their frequent use in practice."

Notice that conditional language is used ("appear to have"). The authors then go on to suggest that more refined studies are warranted. Caveats such as these are standard in journalese, but because they are somewhat clichéd, clinicians usually ignore them. Practitioners reading this might very well come away with the "take home lesson" that antidepressants are ineffective in bipolar depression. In written material, no mention may be made of why, for the reasons I discussed, the results of the study might possibly be invalid.

When some paid "experts" speak at "educational" dinners sponsored by pharmaceutical companies in various contexts, the conditional language is often deemphasized. Conditional phrases are said as a quick aside to leave the speakers a loophole just in case a member of the audience challenges them about overstating their case. Should this happen, the speakers are able to point to the conditional language they used and "remind" the audience that their use of this language indicates that they are not making spurious claims. Most of the time, however, no one in the audience will make such a challenge. The audience is left with a dangling implication that the conclusion is an established fact. Sometimes, however, speakers do not even bother using conditional language at all.

The journey of "established facts" that have not really been established into the common clinical lore is often accelerated by new trainees, who do not have the benefit of the years of clinical experience necessary to know that the new "facts" might be wrong. To use the case above as an example, they will be more likely to avoid the use of antidepressants in bipolar patients and instead use the more expensive brand-name alternatives. Because they have not prescribed them, they have never seen antidepressants work in bipolar patients, so their false belief is maintained. If their teachers have drug company ties, which many do, they might not even hear about the clinical experience of veteran psychiatrists. If they do hear of it, the veteran's experience may be discounted by other teachers as "anecdotal" or "biased."

PSYCHOSOCIAL ISSUES IN BIPOLAR AND UNIPOLAR MAJOR DEPRESSIVE EPISODES

How is the issue of responsiveness to antidepressants in bipolar depression related to the devaluing of psychosocial factors by mental health clinicians? The answer is related to the issue of how a patient feels *after* the resolution of depressed or manic states that were due to the underlying bipolar disorder. When bipolar or unipolar patients return to the normal mood state, they are said to be *euthymic*. However, returning to the euthymic state does not necessarily mean that the patient automatically becomes a happy camper. In the euthymic state, he or she can still feel down just like the rest of us due to situational factors, personality problems, or relationship issues.

If depressive symptoms remain after a clinical depression mostly clears, a question arises. Are the remaining symptoms due to an incomplete response to medication, termed *partial remission* in the DSM, or are they due to psychological factors? They may also be due to a combination of both of these factors. Clues as to the answer to this question can be discovered by a clinician through careful inquiry concerning two additional types of data about the patient.

First, what was the patient's mood *before* he or she ever had had a bipolar mood episode? This is referred to as the patient's *baseline* state. If patients had been chronically unhappy since adolescence because of psychosocial issues, then when they return to baseline after a first bipolar episode, they will still exhibit some depressive symptoms that may not be due to the bipolar disorder. The baseline state of subjects in research studies is almost never specified in a paper, and researchers seldom ask about it at all. "Remission" from the episode is usually defined in studies by a low score on a standardized research interview or self-report measure that asks only about current symptoms.

Second, what is going on in the patients' lives and relationships after they return to the euthymic state? If they have a lot of big problems, then again psychological issues may be the culprit rather than an inadequate medication response. In bipolar patients, psychosocial problems can be horrific because of their behavior when they were manic. Formerly manic patients may have squandered their life savings or had multiple affairs that led to a breakup of their marriages. Being in a *good* mood after events such as these might be the pathological mood state.

Sorting out whether or not residual symptoms are leftovers of a partially remitted major affective episode, are more primarily due to situational and psychological factors, or are due to a combination of the two is extremely difficult because of the huge overlap in symptoms. This is true even if researchers or clinicians take the time to go after the additional history. If they do not, the task is impossible. Obtaining a reliable history of the additional variables takes some time. Researchers almost never bother to do so, and increasingly, neither do clinical psychiatrists.

If the "experts" are successful in convincing clinicians that *all* such symptoms are the result of less than adequate medication response, any residual symptoms the patient has in the euthymic state are more likely to be attributed by the clinician to a poor drug response rather than to psychological factors. These experts then go on to helpfully make suggestions to the clinicians as to what they should do to control the patient's "residual" symptoms. They usually advise substituting the atypical, brand-name antipsychotics or adding them to the antidepressant, thereby increasing the profits of their sponsors.

In November 2007, the drug maker Bristol-Myers Squibb received an FDA indication for its atypical antipsychotic Abilify as an *augmentation* treatment, in combination with antidepressants, for unipolar major depressive episodes. They released the typical army of drug reps and speakers to tout the importance of using their drug for this purpose, since, they said, antidepressants often fail when given by themselves. Again, there was no mention of the possibility that this "failure" of the drug might be related to ongoing psychosocial issues and not due to a patient's partial response to the medication. Unbelievably, the very night after I wrote the earliest draft of this paragraph, I saw a DTC advertisement on national television touting Abilify for depression to the general public using this exact same sales pitch.

At professional get-togethers, these same folks often leave the dangling implication that, since all unhappiness in euthymic unipolar or bipolar patients is "biological" and not "psychological," then *all* patients who are chronically unhappy may have some underlying biological disorder that should therefore be medicated rather than treated with psychotherapy.

Sometimes reps and speakers do not bother to cite any studies at all to make clinical pronouncements. So that the individual who makes such a statement cannot be accused of making things up, once again the statements are usually couched in tentative language. The statements will use conditional words like "may be" or "possibly," or even "probably." However, as these pronouncements are repeated over and over again in throwaway journals and in informal discussions among clinicians, they are often treated as if they are proven facts.

An excellent example of this process concerns the diagnosis of mania in preadolescents, to be discussed in Chapter Seven. I have seen the pronouncement made that, in this population, the normal DSM diagnostic criteria for bipolar disorder in adults do not apply, especially in regards to the duration of the episode necessary to make the diagnosis. In the DSM, manic symptoms must last a week for the diagnosis of mania to be made. For diagnosing major depressive disorder, depressive symptoms must be present almost all day nearly every day for at least two weeks. The reasons for these duration requirements will be discussed in the next chapter.

Several so-called experts have opined that in pediatric bipolar disorder, children may have several mood swings *within a single day*. They also suggest that "atypical" symptoms in children with bipolar disorder should include temper tantrums and explosive irritability. The "terrible twos" has apparently become a mental disorder. No scientific basis for these assertions exists whatsoever; people propagating this point of view usually offer arguments for it that employ circular reasoning. They say that if such children are followed into adulthood, many of them turn out to be bipolar. However, these adult diagnoses are also often highly questionable, for reasons that will also be discussed in the next chapter. Certainly many other simpler explanations for the behavior of temperamental children are possible, and correction of such behavior does not necessarily include the use of highly toxic but brand-name medications.

Drug studies run by pharmaceutical companies are not the only types of studies that can be highly biased. "Empirical" psychotherapy treatment outcome studies are not immune. Following a discussion of this phenomenon, we will look with a fine microscope at the issue of anecdotal evidence.

PROBLEMS AND BIASES IN PSYCHOTHERAPY OUTCOME STUDIES

As I have discussed, psychological processes and reactions are probably one of the two or three most difficult phenomena in nature to study scientifically. We cannot read minds. We have to rely on behavior we can observe and what people tell us is going on in their minds. When you ask people why they do what they do, they may say they do not know. They may lie to you or to themselves. Observers can be and often are deceived.

The Problem of the "False Self"

People do not act the same way in all social contexts. They do not act or speak the same way around a boss that they do when they are alone with a lover. A man's behavior in a strip club is very different than his behavior when he is playing with his children. We have different "faces" or masks that we apply to ourselves in different environments. Not infrequently, these masks are meant to manipulate others to get them to do what we want them to do.

The word *manipulate* has negative connotations, as if it means that we are trying to get others to do our bidding for some nefarious purpose. In truth, we all try to influence one another every day, and sometimes for noble purposes. We want other people to do things with us or for us, and at times we want to do things for them. In order to do this successfully, we must often hide our true feelings and inclinations. We may feign outrage or act warm and sweet when we are feeling some other way entirely. We are all actors. Being able to deceive other members of one's own species under some circumstances has been shown to have survival value in primates.

In dysfunctional families, the masks that members wear are more pervasive. In order for members of such groups to affect other group members, they must often say or do extreme things that under other circumstances they might find unpleasant or even reprehensible. They develop what psychoanalysts have called a *false self.* Other terms for this are *pseudo-self* from family systems pioneer Murray Bowen, and *persona*, from Carl Jung. The behavior they present to the world in a variety of different contexts does not match the way they are really feeling inside. Such behavior becomes habitual and compulsive so that they do not give themselves away accidentally when their guard is down. For this reason, patients in psychotherapy studies may be subconsciously motivated to act out their false self within the study and appear in the final results to be something they are really not.

I never cease to be amazed at how mental health professionals and researchers seem to believe that they really know what is going on in a patient's or a research subject's life based solely on the self-report of the patient, or solely on the reports of the patient's intimates, or even on the reports of people like teachers who observe the behavior of children in only one context that involves thirty other distracting students. If these professionals were asked if they believe that people often act differently in public than they do behind closed doors, they would of course say yes, but they seem to develop amnesia for this fact in discussions and studies.

A patient's family members may be just as motivated to give a distorted view of a patient as is a patient. Parents, for example, may prefer to believe that their child has some sort of mental defect so they do not experience as much of their own covert guilt about their parenting skills. Conversely, some may actually prefer to blame the child's behavior completely on themselves, in order to let their "perfect" child off the hook. Most mental health practitioners do not make home visits to watch patients and family members interact in their natural environment. Even if they did, unless they had a camera operating 24 hours a day as in the movie *The Truman Show*, they could still be deceived.

Flying Blind with Double Blinding

When it comes to psychotherapy treatment outcome studies, we cannot do double-blind placebo-controlled comparisons of two different types of psychotherapy treatments. This is true because, in a sense, the therapist, or more correctly the relationship between the patient and the therapist, *is* the treatment. If the study were to meet the criteria for being double blind, that would mean that the therapists who administer the treatment would have to not know what they were doing.

Of course, they cannot administer psychotherapy without being aware of what techniques they are using. If they could, that would mean that they were incompetent. Not a fair test of a treatment! The fact that the therapy relationship is one of the basic aspects of the treatment also makes placebo or "sham" treatments difficult, because *any* relationship has some effect on an individual. As we have discussed, even small effects may have large consequences.

Does this mean we should give up on evaluating psychotherapy treatment scientifically and rely exclusively on clinical anecdotes? Of course not. Studies are still important. We just have to understand their limitations. Let us look at some of the strategies used in therapy studies, what their limitations are, and how their results are sometimes overstated.

Randomized Clinical Psychotherapy Trials

One strategy used in therapy studies is to compare the outcomes of two different, presumably active types of psychotherapy treatment techniques with each other, rather than with placebo, on similar groups of patients, without the benefit of double blinding. These studies are referred to as *randomized clinical trials*, or RCTs. As we shall see in Chapter Nine, psychotherapy treatment methodology is very diverse, as are psychological theories of maladaptive behavior.

A large number of different *schools* of psychotherapy have different approaches to the understanding of and methodology for changing a patient's repetitive dysfunctional habits. Most of these therapy schools were designed by charismatic and creative individuals who based their ideas on clinical anecdotes, the subject of the next section. These innovators are highly invested emotionally in their own personal theories and want them to look good in comparative psychotherapy outcome studies.

This leads to a so-called *allegiance* effect in RCTs. The preferred psychotherapy school of the researcher is likely to be delivered more enthusiastically and with more rigor to subjects in the study than is the competing therapy treatment. One survey study[12] examined 29 RCT outcome studies that compared one type of therapy to another and found a correlation of .85 between researchers' therapy allegiance and outcome. That is, the researcher's preferred treatment came out ahead 85 percent of the time. Just as in sponsored drug studies, this number is too way high for a significant bias in the studies to be discounted.

When differences are found between two therapies, they are often statistically but not clinically significant. When both groups of therapists who are providing the treatment in the study are equally committed to the paradigms they are delivering, comparative psychotherapy outcome studies almost always result in a tie. In other words, both treatments seem to help, although neither necessarily returns its subject to a state that is equal to known population norms on whatever outcome measures the RCT employs. This phenomenon of different methodologies delivering similar results is very common in all of social science research, such as in studies comparing different methods of teaching reading. In psychotherapy research circles, it is known as the *"dodo bird verdict."* This refers to a character from *Alice in Wonderland*, the dodo bird, who in one passage said, "Everybody has won, and all must have prizes."

Treatment as Usual

Lately, many researchers engaged in psychotherapy RCTs have employed a control group called *treatment as usual* (TAU) that really stacks the deck in favor of their pet psychotherapy school. Lining up practitioners of a different school from the researcher's to act as therapists for a comparison group is often difficult. Additionally, if the researcher were able to do so, the study might not show his or her therapy to be superior to another type. For these reasons, the use of TAU control groups has become almost epidemic in psychotherapy RCTs.

Subjects randomly assigned to the TAU condition, which serves as a comparison group to the group of subjects receiving the researcher's therapy model, are simply released back into the community to get whatever other treatments are already out there. Some may see practitioners from other therapy schools, some may get medications, some may get both, and still others may get neither.

Both the TAU group and the experimental group are followed up at equal time intervals and given all the same outcome measures. The psychotherapy methodology that serves as the investigated treatment always seems to beat TAU.

The reader should understand that within any widely practiced therapy model, both good therapists and bad therapists can be found, just as practicing physicians can be either good or bad psychopharmacologists. For the subjects in the TAU condition who receive treatment, the results of the good clinicians in the community are probably cancelled out by those of the bad ones. TAU subjects may also be seen less frequently. Some are getting no treatment at all. Meanwhile, the experimenter's group is usually getting a lot more individualized attention, which may be the real reason they do better than patients receiving TAU.

The experimenter's therapy is provided by uniformly well-trained and enthusiastic therapists under very well-controlled conditions. The psychotherapy that is provided is applied with rigor and consistency and is scrutinized by other observers through the use of videotapes of the sessions. Therapists who make errors are supervised almost immediately. On top of this, research therapists often have caseloads that are very much smaller than those of folks out in practice, allowing them to spend more time deciding how to approach the clinical issues they face. I cannot recall a single instance in which TAU beat another therapy delivered in such a manner. If it did, I would have to wonder how the experimenter could have possibly accomplished such an unlikely feat.

The Choice of Outcome Measures

Another huge controversy in psychotherapy RCTs is the question of which outcome measures should be used, because the different psychotherapy schools target different aspects of the patient problems under study. What should we measure, exactly? Symptom relief? Whether or not the patients continue to meet criteria for a specific DSM disorder? Whether they stop engaging in chronic repetitive dysfunctional behavior? Whether they experience fewer conflicted emotions? Whether they have improved and more satisfying relationships?

If we pick the last-mentioned outcome, which is the prime focus of most humanistic therapies as opposed to the more symptom-focused therapies such as CBT, how do we measure it? If the subjects in the study say they feel better after they receive a treatment, does that count? Are they even telling the truth?

In their November 1995 issue, *Consumer Reports* published a large survey on the public's experience with psychotherapy. In response to the survey, satisfaction with people's experience was reported widely by those who had been in therapy. Furthermore, longer-term therapy was rated higher than therapy limited in duration by managed care, and satisfaction with psychotherapy was rated about equally by those who had therapy alone and those who were given a combination of therapy and medication.

In surveys of this sort, the question of selection bias arises: whether or not the sample of people polled is representative of the general population. The respondents in this case were almost all middle class and educated, so we have to limit our conclusions to that population rather than the population of the United States as a whole. Nonetheless, the study was the most extensive study of its type on record. Should opinions expressed by patients evaluating psychotherapy outcomes for themselves count as science? Many in the field would say no.

One must consider, however, that psychotherapy is targeted at a patient's *subjective* sense of personal well-being. That is, we want to know whether patients feel better *mentally* about their lives. By this measure, assuming that the survey respondents were being somewhat honest with their answers, we would have to say it should count. A paradox about the "science" of psychotherapy is that we are attempting to be objective about subjectivity, two concepts that are usually defined as antonyms.

Funding Issues

Another big issue for the field concerns which psychotherapy treatment outcome research studies get funded. If a scientist cannot get money for a project, it will rarely get off the ground, because these types of studies are very expensive to mount. Most successful psychotherapy RCTs have employed CBT because of the predominance of this model in professional psychology training programs, and because most CBT treatments aim primarily for symptom reduction, which is relatively easy to measure, rather than personality change, which is not.

The most experienced researchers, which for these reasons tend to be CBT folks, tend to dominate panels that review research proposals for funding agencies such as the NIMH. These people often block funding for studies of alternative or novel treatments. One psychotherapy researcher I know referred to the people on these panels as the "cognitive behavioral mafia." In a manner reminiscent of the arrogance of the psychoanalysts, purveyors of CBT brag that their methods are superior to everyone else's because they have the most successful RCTs, while they are the very ones preventing other models from ever being studied.

Problems with Generalizability of Study Results

Another big problem with all psychotherapy RCTs is that most studies require that the subject population be *homogeneous*, meaning that the subjects in the study must be very similar in the nature and severity of the disorder they exhibit. This requirement means that patients who have more than one DSM disorder or psychological problem are often excluded from studies. Most patients seen in practice, at least by psychiatrists, have more than one disorder *(co-morbidity)*. This fact alone limits what is termed the *generalizability* of the study's finding. We do not know from a study using patients who have only one disorder if the treatment employed in the study would work as well with patients who have multiple problems.

Because studies need subjects who will stick with the treatment until the end of the research project, some subjects who have certain characteristics that are common in clinical practice tend to be excluded. This problem further limits the generalizability of the study. For instance, most studies of treatments for depression exclude patients who are suicidal. They are excluded because they are likely during the course of the study to have a crisis requiring hospitalization, which if necessary would add a second kind of treatment. Most studies must employ only one treatment, because if the study were contaminated by other treatments, it would end up comparing apples to oranges. On the other hand, methinks suicidality is an extremely important characteristic to study. Nonetheless, suicidal patients are left out of most RCTs, including drug studies.

Another problem with RCTs is that many subjects drop out of a study or are removed from a study as it proceeds because they do not completely cooperate with the treatment in some way. CBT studies, as do many others, tend to have a fairly high dropout rate. What this usually means is that data from subjects with more severe or intractable cases of any disorder, or with significant personality issues, are not included in the final data. Furthermore, the subjects who end up completing the study are usually the most motivated to change, and would therefore be expected to do better than those who lack this motivation. This all makes the treatment method look much better than it would be if it were employed in a typical clinical practice setting.

CBT often includes homework assignments that patients must agree to carry out in between therapy sessions. Those subjects who do not complete the assignments, which are presumed to be integral to the treatment, would be assumed for that reason to benefit far less from the treatment than those subjects who do. In clinical experience, failure to complete homework assignments is the norm rather than the exception. CBT researchers are therefore affected by yet another bias. In this case they prefer highly motivated subjects over others. This consideration probably enters into how they select their subjects prior to randomization. This factor would again inflate the apparent efficacy of the treatment.

A great example of this problem can be seen with treatment studies of patients who have obsessive-compulsive disorder, such as those who engage in compulsive hand washing. Textbooks make the psychotherapy treatment of these highly impaired individuals sound so easy. The CBT treatment is glibly summarized as *exposure* and *response prevention*. If the compulsive hand washers are exposed to situations in which they feel that their hands are dirty and are prevented from washing their hands for an extended period of time, they get better. The treatment method really is effective, but only if the patient cooperates.

The problem is this: I do not suppose that many lay readers of this book have ever tried to get a person with a severe compulsion to *not* engage in it for an extended period of time. Well, I have. Obsessive-compulsive disorder is not called that for nothing. Such patients can hardly stand to stop for even a few minutes. Unless you can get the patient to agree to let a therapist literally tie his or her hands for a few days, he or she *will* engage in hand washing, and the treatment definitely will not work. Somehow published efficacy studies always seem to give this problem short shrift.

Treatment Manuals

Another big issue in psychotherapy outcome studies is that, in comparing different treatments for different behavioral problems, researchers need to have some way of knowing that all the therapists employed in the study are doing mostly the same things. In early psychotherapy studies, the methods section of a journal report might say that such and such number of patients was "given psychoanalytic therapy," with no description of what the therapists actually did. This was clearly unacceptable.

The solution to this problem that has been employed is the use of treatment manuals, as well as manuals that measure the study therapists' competence in and their adherence to the treatment paradigm. Treatment and adherence manuals specify exactly what the therapist should be doing under a variety of circumstances. Tapes of psychotherapy sessions of patients in the studies are reviewed to make sure that the therapists are employing the same interventions. A "rater" will count the times the therapist did the right thing and the times the therapist strayed from the procedures specified in the manual. This process ensures that all patients are getting approximately the same treatment.

Interestingly, training CBT therapists so that they are consistent in sticking to the dictates of a CBT treatment manual can take a whole year, in spite of the fact that they have already been trained in CBT. This problem shows up for other types of psychotherapy as well. Why is this? In practice, psychotherapy cannot always be guided by a cookbook, and a cookbook is basically what a therapy treatment manual is. As I have mentioned, similar patients can respond very differently to similar interventions. A good therapist has to be flexible and employ a variety of different strategies in ways that are tailored to the proclivities and sensitivities of each patient. Generic interventions may not only fail to work, but they may also backfire and make matters worse. Verbal interventions must often be phrased differently to different patients to reduce the patient's defensiveness.

Treatment and adherence manuals take away some of this flexibility, so that the therapy as performed in an RCT is not always similar to the way that clinicians out in the field practice it. This further limits the generalizability of the study results. Unfortunately, avoiding the use of such manuals also limits the usefulness of the results of the study, because without the manuals no one would be able to know exactly what the subjects were getting from the therapist.

Creating treatment manuals can itself be a daunting task. I heard a respected researcher tell a group of other researchers that his team was having trouble designing such a manual because the founder of the treatment they wanted to study was observed to perform psychotherapy completely differently than his own wife, who supposedly was a practitioner of the same model of therapy.

Process Research

Besides RCTs, there is another form of "empirical" psychotherapy treatment research called *process research*. Psychotherapy from any individual school employs a wide variety of different interventions. Some of these interventions may be essential, others sometimes helpful and sometimes not, and still others completely unnecessary or even counterproductive. One might say that therapies take a shotgun approach to changing patient behavior, cognitions, and feelings. Discovering which interventions are the active ingredients of the therapy helps any treatment plan to be more efficient and probably more effective.

One way to study this is to watch or listen to therapy sessions, or read transcripts of them, to try to discern what happens during and right after the various interventions performed by the therapist. These sessions can then be compared to sessions with other patients and therapists to see what interventions, and under what circumstances and for which types of patients, seem to produce the best results. Subjects and therapists can also be asked to look at the tapes and comment about what was going through their minds at certain times during the session. Studies that employ these techniques are called process studies because they look at the process of what happens during interchanges between patients and therapists. Much of today's psychotherapy research employs this method.

Psychotherapy researchers who do process studies have complained for years that clinicians seem to ignore their work. I think I understand why that happens. The results of most of their studies are either somewhat trivial, or they show things that experienced therapists already know. Therefore, most practicing therapists do not read them because they are not worth their time. Again, this does not mean that such studies should not be done. It is helpful to have evidence that what we think we know is actually true. Still, more important readings are plentiful, and clinicians' time is limited.

As an example, one psychology intern I worked with published an excellent study that showed that, in instances when patients become suddenly silent during a therapy session, the silence can mean completely different things depending on other factors. It might mean, for example, that patients are reflecting on what the therapist has just said because it was new and interesting to them, but it could also mean they are offended by what the therapist has said. When the intern asked me what I thought of the study, I sort of grimaced. It was a good study, but to me it was psychotherapy 101. Teasing apart, the different meanings of patient silences is part of basic psychoanalytically oriented psychotherapy training.

I recall a discussion I had with a psychotherapy researcher about why most studies seem to be about either trivial or already well-known aspects of psychotherapy. Surely there must be more important or controversial aspects of psychotherapy to look at. In response, he told me the old joke about the drunk searching for his lost keys under a lamp post at night. A helpful passerby asks the drunk if he had dropped his keys under the post. The drunk replies that, no, he had lost them half a block away. Then why, asks the passerby, was he looking where he was looking? "Because that is where the light is," the drunk replies.

In other words, researchers do studies that are easy to design and implement from a scientific standpoint so they can author more papers and be more widely published. In many academic centers, faculty members must either publish or perish. Studies examining more important or controversial aspects of psychotherapy—usually the softer humanistic and family relationship issues—are much more difficult to do.

So how do we get to the bottom of the more complex, difficult, and hidden workings of the human mind? The answer is that we have to employ, in addition to scientific studies, clinical anecdotes. They too have obvious limitations, but we need to combine all sources of data in any type of psychological science to get to the truth.

ANECDOTAL EVIDENCE: THE GOOD, THE BAD, AND THE UGLY

Anecdotal evidence in medicine is often misleadingly defined as evidence based on only one clinician's personal experience with a treatment or diagnosis in question. If that is the standard that is to be used, clearly many reasons exist to question the validity of inferences drawn from these experiences. Individuals are well known to have various biases that color their observations and the conclusions they draw from them. They may have blind spots because of their own emotional conflicts. They may ignore evidence that is contradictory to their point of view. Their observations may be limited by their pet theories about the phenomena in question. They may be seeing unusual cases that are not representative of more "typical" cases in one way or another: a so-called *selection bias*.

An obvious case of selection bias was illustrated by a statement I heard made at a conference by a family therapy pioneer, the late Jay Haley. I had always admired Mr. Haley for many of his fascinating and utilitarian ideas and observations. However, in this case he betrayed some ignorance. He stated that he did not believe antidepressant drugs were ever effective because none of the patients referred to him had ever responded to them. Of course, his being a well-known family therapist who did not believe in medication had a tremendous effect on exactly who would be referred to him. Not everyone does respond to drug treatment. Anyone who *had* responded to an antidepressant would, in all probability, rarely if ever darken his door. Hence, with his sample, he would be misled into thinking that the medicines were not effective for anybody. This form of bias is very common and can be quite subtle. For example, it can affect one's beliefs about such matters as racial stereotypes or a determination of how trustworthy members of a city's police department are.

Descriptions versus Conclusions

Do these types of biases invalidate all clinical experience? Hardly. First of all, we have to distinguish between the descriptions of the actual events contained within specific anecdotes and the *conclusions* or inferences that are drawn from these events. Let us examine the descriptions of what actually happened. A specific anecdote may be accurately observed and described, or not so accurately. If important details are altered or left out entirely, the anecdote may indeed be worthless. However, the exact same thing can be said about empirical studies.

Important details may not even be known to an observer. With observations of family behavior within a practitioner's or researcher's office, important information is almost always hidden. In addition to the fact that one does not see the whole picture in any single context, there is also a basic problem inherent in the nature of interactions between intimates. With verbal behavior, for instance, linguists refer to a quality called *ellipsis*. What this means is that in conversations among people who have known each other for a while, certain information is not spelled out verbally because the other person already knows it. Strangers such as therapists who are listening in and who have not been privy to these prior experiences may think they know what the family is talking about, but they may in reality be completely clueless.

In my talks to trainees, I often show a videotape of a grown woman bitterly attacking her father because he made her do chores when she was a teenager. Poor dear, she had to do chores. How terrible! Most viewers feel sorry for the gentleman until I let them know that one of her "chores" was providing her father with sexual release when he was between wives. Although neither the woman nor her father ever mentions this specifically on the tape, if the observer knows this fact, the real subject of the conversation becomes more and more clear as the session progresses.

Let us now consider the separate issue of conclusions that are drawn from anecdotes, as opposed to their description. The questions raised by an accurately described clinical observation can be quite valid, but the answers inferred from it can be completely wrong. Conclusions based on clinical "anecdotes" exist on a continuum from relatively accurate ones to those that are extremely biased to those that are based on spectacular inferential or logical leaps of faith.

Relatively unbiased clinical conclusions based on anecdotes by mental health professionals have many things in common:

1. They are based on a sample that one has a reasonable expectation is at least somewhat representative of a larger population.
2. They use, not just the practitioner's observations, but also the observations of other professionals whom one knows to be reliable and open-minded. These clinicians should also be ones known to take the time with their patients that is necessary to take a complete history.
3. They make use of other informants besides the patient when possible.
4. They take into consideration that people and their family members behave quite differently behind closed doors than they do in public, and therefore if at all possible include observations of patient behavior when patients are *unaware that they are being observed*.
5. They are based on longitudinal observations. That is, the patients on whom conclusions are based have been seen on multiple occasions over an extended period of time.
6. They are not contradicted by commonly observed examples of behavior in everyday life related to the behavior in question.
7. The person proposing the conclusion acknowledges potential biases, such as a financial stake in a certain drug or allegiance to a specific school of therapy, and acknowledges his or her limitations. What former president of the Society of Clinical Psychology, Gerald C. Davison, calls "ex cathedra statements based upon flimsy and subjective evidence,"[13] a hallmark of some psychotherapy gurus, are always highly suspicious. In fact, charlatans are relatively easy to spot. Their attitude is, "Trust me and just believe that my methods are highly effective." According to Neil Jacobson,[14] false prophets show no humility or doubt, exhibit an indifference to independent tests, and have a tendency to sidestep challenges. I give several examples throughout this book of so-called experts sidestepping questions, and will mention another shortly.
8. The conclusions reached should lead to predictions of patient behavior under certain circumstances that prove to be accurate in a significant number of cases. This is called *predictive validity*. Of course, human behavior being as unpredictable as it is, at times

the predictions will not be completely accurate even if the conclusions are valid, and so this fact must also be taken into account.

9. Conclusions based on anecdotes about treatment efficacy or the reasons for certain observed behavior should consider several alternate possible explanations for the observations. If several explanations are possible, one must make a judgment about which ones are more likely and which are less likely based not on the anecdote alone, but on *all* sources of data available. These sources include empirical studies, but also include observations from everyday life, as well as material seen in some relatively reliable media such as reputable newspapers.

Now of course stories in the media may also not tell the whole story or be biased, so one needs to realize again that one can be fooled, and take this into account as well. I used to believe the common myth, for example, that in nature under certain conditions the animals called lemmings would follow each other off a cliff and commit mass suicide. I was surprised when I learned that this was untrue because I had as a child in 1958 seen a film clip of said mass suicide that was part of a Disney "True Life Adventure" nature movie called *White Wilderness*. I later learned that, because the Disney crew could not find a real example, they had from behind the scenes driven the group of lemmings off the cliff for the cameras.

On the other hand, many people believe that men have never been to the moon and that films of the moon landings were made in a movie studio using special effects. I must say, I tend to believe that those film clips are real, but few know for certain.

10. If other anecdotes about similar patients and treatments seem to contradict the conclusions based on a given anecdote, an attempt should be made to account for this difference. As an illustration of this point and an example of the "quick step side step," I heard an expert present new evidence from neuroscience that certain capabilities of which human brains are capable seem to develop only at certain times during early childhood development. This brain development could be adversely affected by a baby's early social environment. Of course, that is somewhat true. As psychoanalysts will, however, the expert went on to conclude that if the adverse early experiences had taken place, the child had no chance of growing up to be normal. I raised my hand and asked about those children who come from horribly adverse backgrounds, are adopted away at an age past the alleged crucial developmental time, and yet still turn out wonderfully. The expert then changed the subject without ever addressing my question.

Listening to my fellow psychiatrists, I can often spot problems with conclusions drawn from clinical anecdotes that, because of my own anecdotal experiences, tell me that their anecdote may be invalid and that I need to use other data besides theirs to form an opinion. One of the most common examples of such a problem is described in the next section.

Once a Diagnosis, Always the Diagnosis

As a clinician as well as the director of a psychiatric training program, I have had many opportunities to observe the same patient in a variety of contexts at different times. As a prime example, I worked for a time in a psychiatric emergency room in Memphis, from which many patients were referred for psychiatric hospitalization. After having evaluated a patient in the ER, I would later see the same patient in the hospital on weekends, when I was covering a service for the doctors who were in charge of the patient in the new setting. I would review the patient's chart for the events and subsequent evaluations that had occurred since admission. One thing I witnessed time and time again, and not just with trainees but also with the attending faculty, was quite striking.

In the ER, some patients looked very depressed and showed all the *signs* (observed characteristics) and complained of all the symptoms of clinical major depressive disorder. Their movements and speech were slow (*psychomotor retardation*), and they complained of chronic and persistent changes in appetite, sleep, pleasure, energy, and concentration. Since they seemed to meet all of the necessary DSM criteria, the diagnosis of major depressive disorder was therefore made by my resident, and I concurred.

However, in many cases in which I saw the patient in the hospital the very next day, or heard a description of the patient's behavior on the ward by the nurses on the day following admission, an entirely different picture emerged. The patient was observed to be actively socializing with other patients, friendly and talkative on approach, speaking with normal rate and volume, sleeping on hourly bed checks (although he or she often had been given a sedative), and eating 100 percent of served meals. These observations were seen right from the start of the hospitalization on nurse's note after nurse's note in the chart.

One major characteristic that distinguishes true major depressive disorder from other types of depression is that its symptoms do not evaporate overnight, nor do they disappear merely because of a change of venue for the patient. They persist and are present in all environmental contexts. They can get to the point where a patient could win the lottery but not crack a smile.

Clearly, everyone's initial diagnostic impression of these patients, including my own, was incorrect. Surprisingly, the patients' diagnosis was never changed during the entire course of their hospitalization. Their admission and discharge diagnoses were identical. Furthermore, they had been given treatments that patients who actually had major depression would be given.

Were my observations of this phenomenon biased in some way? Perhaps not changing a diagnosis in the light of new and conflicting information was something peculiar to doctors practicing in academic settings or only those practicing in Memphis, the city in which I was located. Possible, but not likely. How do I know? Well, in over thirty years of practice, I have had the opportunity to review medical records all over the United States of patients who had been psychiatrically hospitalized.

The hospital progress notes written by psychiatrists were often quite uninformative, because they would not describe the patient's behavior on the ward after admission. I, being a contrarian, would take a look instead at the nurses' notes. There, the patient's behavior on the ward was described in detail. The same problem I had observed was obviously occurring frequently all over the country. The long-term process of seeing multiple records from multiple observers from multiple places multiple times turns an "anecdote" into reasonably unbiased "data."

Paradoxically, the fact that initial diagnoses are often not revised even in the presence of evidence that they are wrong affects double-blind placebo-controlled studies as much if not more than it does clinical observations. Particularly in drug studies, subjects are generally not seen daily nor over a period of time longer than several weeks so that diagnostic errors might become apparent. Social histories are not taken, nor are efforts made to gain the trust of subjects who might initially have reasons to avoid being truthful. Nonetheless, in most studies, once the diagnosis is made, it is assumed to be correct for the rest of the study. If there are any such errors, they are assumed to fall equally between the experimental groups and the controls, thereby canceling one another out. Unfortunately, there is no way to test if the experimental and control groups are in reality equivalent in this respect.

Another common problem related to the "once a diagnosis, always a diagnosis" phenomenon is that once patients are given a diagnosis, they can carry it for the rest of their lives even if it is entirely wrong. The incorrect diagnoses can then hound the patients, making their lives more difficult in a variety of ways. Many mental health providers rely on the diagnoses and treatments rendered by other clinicians who have treated the patient earlier. I teach my residents that, while they should take into account previous diagnoses and treatments in their initial evaluations, they should nonetheless do a complete evaluation of the patient on their own, and form their own opinion.

The former chairman of my department, Neil Edwards, used to tell residents that the evaluation of each patient new to a clinician should take into account two different possibilities: first, that any prior clinician was competent, thorough, and correct, and second, that the prior clinician was none of these things. For the oral psychiatry board exam, examiners are supposed to insist that the examinee do his or her own exam and not rely entirely on previous diagnoses.

Even before managed care began to eat away at physicians' income and led many to start seeing more and more patients in less and less time, clinicians frequently relied on earlier evaluations and diagnoses. If a patient was diagnosed as schizophrenic, for example, they would keep that diagnosis for a very long time. I recall one patient who, before commitment laws were altered to preclude indefinite involuntary hospitalization, had been institutionalized for thirty years with that diagnosis. Finally, one astute clinician had the forethought to do his own complete evaluation and discovered that the patient had the more easily treatable condition of bipolar disorder. She was placed on lithium, to which she responded well, and was discharged.

Although she never had another psychotic episode, she still had significant psychological problems. These were almost all due to the fact that she had been institutionalized for thirty years and no longer knew how to negotiate life on the outside. The adjustment to a more "normal" life was exceedingly difficult for her. This behavioral problem, by the way, had absolutely nothing to do with her bipolar disorder per se.

Clearly a correct diagnosis, even in an age when we do not know the real causes of many psychiatric syndromes, is important. Wrong diagnoses can have horrendous consequences for patients. The rather loose ways in which psychiatric diagnoses are often made nowadays, including the neglect of the most important psychosocial factors creating a patient's misery, is the subject of the next chapter.

7

Diagnonsense

As I have discussed, a major strategy through which managed care has turned much of psychiatric practice into mangled care is the provision of financial incentives for psychiatrists to spend far less time with patients per visit than they did in the past, even when they are only doing *medication management* and not psychotherapy. Because they are being paid so much less per patient, they try to see more and more patients per hour. In public psychiatry, such as that practiced in community mental health centers, government and public support has dwindled to such an extent in the face of expanding numbers of indigent and uninsured patients that, in order for a clinician to provide any care at all, the brief amount of time a patient visit must last is literally specified in a clinician's employment contract.

A typical psychiatrist's follow-up visit for a medication check is scheduled for about 10 to 15 minutes. If a patient has been stable on his or her medication for a while and psychological or social problems are not a major contributing factor in producing the patient's symptomatology, 10 minutes may be more than sufficient. Unfortunately, the problems of many patients in psychiatric treatment are a bit more complicated. Teasing out the psychological factors influencing the patient's presentation from the more biological ones, the latter in general being far more responsive to medications, takes much more time. When a psychiatrist does not take the time to do this properly, a misdiagnosis is the not-too-infrequent consequence.

FOCUSING ONLY ON SYMPTOMS

Rather than taking extra time during a medication check, a psychiatrist may only ask about the state of the patient's symptoms since the previous visit, and not inquire about any changes in the patient's problematic relationships or in the level of environmental stressors. As we shall see, a good assessment of the diagnostic significance and treatment implications of any psychiatric symptom requires an understanding of the entire psychological *context* in which the symptom occurs. A good *case formulation* involves the evaluation of all biological, psychological, and social factors affecting the patient's outward presentation.

The manner in which requests for treatment authorizations are structured by managed care companies has also been a factor in leading many clinicians to focus solely on a patient's symptoms rather than on either the disorder that causes the symptoms or, God forbid, the whole person who is experiencing the symptoms. These treatment authorizations are based almost entirely on the patient's superficial symptoms and the improvement thereof rather than on a complete case formulation. Insurance companies brag that this means that they are "problem and solution" oriented. As a colleague named David Reiss once put it, many modern psychiatrists act as if they are treating neurotransmitters in a test tube rather than in a patient.

Some unscrupulous psychiatrists do not even spend 10 or 15 minutes per follow-up visit with a patient after their initial evaluation. One hospital psychiatrist in my community was sarcastically rumored to be a practitioner of "wave therapy." Wave therapy on an inpatient unit is said to consist of a doctor saying hello to a patient and then waving goodbye while turning away and saying hello to another patient. Unfortunately, this tongue-in-cheek description was not much of an exaggeration, nor was this doctor's modus operandi all that unusual. Some psychiatrists use masters-level social workers to funnel information to them, and even let them write prescriptions, which the psychiatrist then signs with minimal oversight.

Symptom Focus and the Use of Psychiatric Hospitalization

Insurance companies now require that psychiatric patients be seen every day while hospitalized, under the theory that if someone is sick enough to be in the hospital, he or she must be in need of a doctor's frequent attention. With psychiatric patients, this theory is not especially true, because psychiatric medications usually take many days to work, and the patient's condition may change very little from one day to the next. The nursing staff can easily alert the doctor to the necessity of a visit in the interim. When I was in practice in the 1970s, I saw my hospitalized patients only three times per week, and I discharged them faster on the average than any other psychiatrist I knew.

While paradoxically this policy of managed care allows the doctors to run up the patient's bill by having more frequent examinations than necessary, my suspicion is that the policy was originally meant to inconvenience doctors so they would be less inclined to hospitalize patients with the resultant high costs, even though they could see more patients per hour in the hospital than they could in the office and therefore make more money. The managed care companies instituted policies designed, successfully, to limit hospital patient stays to just a few days, often less time than it takes for psychiatric medications to improve the patient's disorder in any meaningful way.

In order to make more money with such frequent patient turnover, psychiatrists and hospitals became increasingly creative in devising reasons to hospitalize patients instead of treating them in an office setting. One way to keep their census of hospitalized patient high is by turning common behavioral problems into more severe "biological" psychiatric disorders such as bipolar disorder through creative diagnostic techniques.

This goal can best be accomplished by ignoring the psychological, social, and temporal context behind patients' symptoms and merely accepting patient reports about them at face value. So that the reader understands how this practice can "upgrade" a patient's psychological problems to a more serious disorder, I will first discuss the elements of a good psychiatric history. If you are already familiar with these elements, please feel free to skip to the subsection entitled "Psychological Testing."

THE PSYCHIATRIC HISTORY

When it comes to time spent with a patient, follow-up visits are one thing, but the patient's initial evaluation is something else entirely. A good psychiatric diagnostic interview takes at a minimum 45 minutes because it necessitates gathering enough information to make a good case formulation. This involves the assessment of the development over time of *all* biological, psychological, and social factors affecting the patient's mental state. Many psychiatrists, and not just those who are trying to artificially inflate their hospitalized patient census, have opted or have been forced by their employers to schedule new patients for only 30 minutes, with no time allotted in between patients to write notes, return phone calls, or even go to the restroom. In such a situation, clinicians look for additional shortcuts.

A good psychiatric history consists of the patient's complaint, a detailed history of the nature and time course of his or her current symptoms, inquiries about any and all other possible symptoms that the patient's presentation might suggest, an exhaustive history of any earlier psychiatric complaints or treatment, the incidence of any history of psychiatric problems in the patient's blood relatives, information about medical problems and substance abuse, and an examination of the patient's current mental state. Importantly, it should also include a history of the patient's current living situation, relationships, early family experiences, education, and occupational functioning. This latter part of the exam is often termed a *social history.*

Time can be saved by cutting corners on the elicitation of the patient's symptom profile and by avoiding taking a social history altogether. The problem with this approach is that a given symptom, depending on other factors, may be seen in a variety of different diagnoses. Particular symptoms can also appear quite similar to other, completely different symptoms. An example of a symptom that is seen in a variety of very different conditions is irritability. Depending on its context and pervasiveness, it can be a symptom of a personality disorder, depression, mania, an ongoing interpersonal dispute with an intimate, or just having a bad day for no particular reason at all.

An example of two symptoms that are extremely similar but whose differentiation is important is rumination, seen in depression, and obsessions, which are seen in obsessive-compulsive disorder. Ruminating consists of worrying over and over again about a wide variety of different but realistic everyday concerns, such as whether one will be able to pay all the bills. An obsession is a single thought or small group of thoughts that comes to a person unbidden and stays in his or her mind for a long time, repeating over and over. An obsession generally concerns something clearly unrealistic, such as thoughts of being contaminated by everyday germs. The evaluating clinician must take time to tease out the particulars in order to make this kind of differentiation.

Making the diagnosis of personality problems is especially time consuming, because teasing out subtle differences in traits is particularly important. For instance, the trait of being mistrustful or paranoid is a prime symptom of three different personality disorders. What determines to which of these three disorders the trait should be assigned is the reason for the mistrust. In paranoid personality disorder, the individual is mistrustful because he thinks he is special in some way and that others want something from him, or he just thinks everyone is untrustworthy even when he has significant evidence to the contrary. In BPD, patients mistrust others initially because they have been frequently betrayed by people whom they were supposed to trust. In avoidant personality disorder, patients mistrust others because they are afraid that others will judge them harshly or that they will look foolish. Since personality disorders respond mostly to psychotherapy rather than medication, many psychiatrists do not even bother to try to diagnose them at all.

The importance of the social history can be illustrated by a case of a hypothetical female patient coming to see a doctor complaining of depression. Let us say that her symptom profile is consistent with a major depressive disorder, and so the doctor prescribes an antidepressant medication for her. She comes back in a month saying she is no better, so the doctor increases the dose. After another month of nonresponse, he changes the medication to a different antidepressant agent, but the patient is still no better. However, the patient had neglected to tell the doctor that her husband is beating her on a regular basis right in front of her children. She has carefully hidden her bruises.

A patient may not tell doctors about such beatings for a number of reasons. The doctor may not have asked, so she might assume that this fact was not important for him to know. She might not trust the doctor, because she has met him only once or twice and she may previously have had many confidences betrayed by persons in authority. She may be afraid that if her husband finds out that she told the doctor that the abuse might get worse, or that she will be thrown out on the street. She may be afraid that she would be unable to support herself and her children if he went to jail, or that her children might be taken away from her. She also might be ashamed that she cannot make herself leave the marriage. She therefore hides the truth.

In any event, a treatment failure in such a case is probably not due to unresponsiveness to medication per se. It may occur because her symptoms are entirely reactive to the abuse and would go away on their own if the abuse stopped. Even if she has been correctly diagnosed, a good response to medication alone is highly unlikely if the beatings continue.

In a good psychiatric diagnostic interview, the clinician must act like an investigative news reporter interviewing a politician. The interviewer must be able to sense when his or her questions are being either evaded, sidestepped, or misunderstood by a patient, and follow-up questions must be asked to clarify the situation. The interviewer should also be aware of statements that patients make under their breath or in passing that call into question a diagnosis the clinician is considering. Details are extremely important. Good follow-up questions, like those of a good newsman, include when, where, under what circumstances, why, how, and how long.

Psychological Testing

Some psychologists and psychiatrists make use of psychological testing to make a diagnosis in place of performing a complete interview. The problem with relying exclusively on tests is twofold. First, they are unable to make subtle distinctions about symptoms and character traits. Making these distinctions, as mentioned, may require follow-up questions to see if the patient understood exactly what the test questions are trying to get at. Follow-up questions are impossible in a testing situation because they require a sophisticated understanding of how the patient may have initially responded to a test item.

Second, a clinician can learn a lot about patients by observing *how* they answer a question, the look on their faces as they do so, and what information they seem to omit. These data are lost during testing. In my opinion, except in those cases in which doctors have a need to find and delineate ill-defined and subtle neurological impairments as might be seen in early Alzheimer's disease, expensive psychological testing is usually unnecessary.

I picked up on this point during my residency. When we ordered psychological testing on a patient, one of the faculty psychologists would come back in a day or two with an amazingly detailed report about the end results. He was able to make fine diagnostic distinctions and identify character traits that I had not picked up during my beginner's psychiatric history and mental status exam. I was extremely impressed by the kinds of information psychological testing seemed capable of producing.

When I started a hospital job after completing residency, I had a completely different experience with testing. I would pose a question to the psychologists such as "Is this patient's clinical picture more consistent with acute schizophrenia or mania?" The psychologists would do the exact same tests that the academic psychologist had done. When the report came back, it would say that the patient had either acute schizophrenia or acute mania. I knew that already. The question I had asked the psychologists in the first place was about which one of these two diagnoses it was most likely to be. I experienced this sort of result with psychological testing again and again.

I became by this time very disappointed in the utility of psychological testing, and for a while I just could not understand the immeasurable difference in the reports of the academic psychologist and the practicing psychologists. Then it hit me. I remembered something the academic psychologist had told me in passing. In addition to the tests, he spent one to two hours interviewing the patients.

Is a Symptom Significant?

Of course, even spending the time necessary to do a complete diagnostic interview is no guarantee that it will be done right. A common beginner's mistake during a trainee's initial patient evaluations is not appreciating that sometimes a patient is actually answering a different question from the one the doctor thinks he or she has asked. For example, the trainee may ask a depressed woman about sleep disturbances *during* a depressive episode, and think the patient understands that, when the patient actually thinks the doctor wants to know whether or not she has *ever* had a sleep disturbance. This is an extremely important distinction. Sleep problems can be symptoms of a variety of different diagnoses, including different types of depression, or they may be a symptom of some sort of normal reaction to events in the patient's life.

To qualify for the diagnosis *major depressive disorder*, the sleep problem has to occur *only* during the episode. If a patient *always* has trouble sleeping, then the doctor is not supposed to count the symptom toward the required number of symptoms necessary to make the diagnosis, unless the sleep problem gets *worse* during the depressive episodes. Making a correct diagnosis is important not only for its own sake, but also in treatment considerations. For example, certain types of depression do not respond as well as others to certain antidepressants. I have already mentioned a woman who was institutionalized for years because of a misdiagnosis of schizophrenia.

Particularly in distinguishing mood disorders from one another and from other diagnoses, the time course of the symptoms is of crucial relevance. If it is not elicited correctly, the correct diagnosis will be missed. Most beginners do not take the time necessary to understand the entire time course of each of the patient's symptoms.

Another similar consideration in making a mood disorder diagnosis is that all of the symptoms have to be present *at the same time.* If you had a poor appetite two weeks ago but it is really hearty right now, and today, unlike two weeks ago, you are feeling lethargic, the two symptoms cannot both be counted toward the diagnosis of the same depressive episode.

Still another important distinction in mood disorder diagnosis is the pervasiveness of a symptom. For major depression, the DSM requires that symptoms be present nearly all day nearly every day for at least two weeks. The two-week period is arbitrary but was put in the DSM to rule out depressive reactions to major environmental stressors that take place only in the presence of the stressor. In another type of depression, *dysthymia,* the symptoms can come and go, but they should be present about half the time for at least two *years.*

The tendency to overdiagnose major depression at the expense of dysthymia has contributed to turning psychiatrists' attention away from psychosocial factors contributing to the patient's condition, such as discordant family interactions, in favor solely of biological factors. Dysthymia tends to involve the thinking part of the brain, the *cortex,* more than does major depressive disorder, which primarily involves the brain's more primitive part called the *limbic system.* Major depression tends to be more amenable to medication than it is to psychotherapy, particularly if it is severe. Dysthymic depressions, on the other hand, tend to respond better to psychotherapy and are more often triggered by chronic problematic relationships with intimates.

Of course, there is considerable overlap between the symptoms of major depression, either of the unipolar or the bipolar varieties, and dysthymia, because all parts of the brain have a multitude of connections to all other parts. A patient can also develop a major depression (or a manic episode) on top of a preexisting dysthymia. This is referred to as a *double depression.* Dysthymia is in fact a risk factor for the more limbic form of depression, again most likely because of all those brain connections between the two parts of the brain. The distinction between these various forms of depression has strong treatment implications.

Many psychiatrists, in order to see more patients in less time, continue to make the beginner's mistakes. They do not probe the patient's answers to see if, first, the patient really understood the question being asked, and second, if the symptom reported fits the profile for major depression or the profile for dysthymia. This neglect of the nature and psychological and social context of psychiatric symptoms is also inherent in the use of another unconscionable diagnostic shortcut, the *symptom checklist*.

Symptom Checklists

Symptom checklists are often given to patients to fill out before they are seen by the clinician, and the clinician then does a rather cursory interview based almost entirely on the patients' answers to the questionnaire. This sort of shortcut may also be used in the evaluation of subjects in research projects. The clinician or researcher does not necessarily make sure that the patient who does or does not endorse a symptom appreciates the importance of the subtleties of where, how, and in what time frame the symptom should be present to be useful in making a particular diagnosis. In office practice, the checklist is usually made up by the clinician using some sort of research tool as a reference.

The research tools or treatment outcome measures that clinicians use as a reference are either clinical interviews that rigidly follow a series of clinical questions or observations, or they are "self-report" instruments on which the patient answers a series of questions about certain symptoms and their severity. Many of these instruments were never designed to be used to make a diagnosis, but only to measure changes in symptom severity in patients already diagnosed by other means, or to force a clinician or researcher to inquire about symptoms or variables about which he or she might forget to ask.

For instance, a research interview for evaluating marital conflict might turn up information about physical abuse that a female subject might not volunteer if she were asked about abuse in general. The checklist might specifically ask her if she has been pushed, kicked, or slapped. The subject who has been abused may not consider those acts to be abuse, and so may not mention them unless asked about them by name.

To show how symptom checklists are poor diagnostic tools by themselves, allow me to describe their use in depressed patients. In studies of depression, two of the more commonly used symptom checklists are the self-administered Beck Depression Inventory and the clinician-administered Hamilton Depression Rating Scale. None of the items on either scale ask precisely how long or under what circumstances any given depressive symptom has been present, so they do not clearly differentiate patients with major depressive disorder from patients with dysthymia.

Checklists usually ask whether or not certain symptoms are present and then ask the interviewer or the subject to rate the severity of the symptoms. Severity ratings are usually made using a *Likert Scale*, a scale of 0 to 5 or 7 in which a 0 means the symptom is absent and the highest number means the symptom is most severe. Alternately, each symptom may be rated using what are called *anchor points*. Anchor points are more detailed descriptions of what each given rating of a symptom should mean.

In mania, a very commonly used instrument is the *Young Mania Rating Scale*,[1] used to evaluate the current presence or absence of symptoms of mania and their severity. It its original form, it is supposed to be administered by a researcher and is said to take 15 to 30 minutes to go through. The first symptom listed is "elevated mood." A 0 rating means that this symptom is absent, while a rating of 2 means the presence of subjective mood elevation characterized by such things as optimism and cheerfulness. A rating of 4 means that the patient exhibits euphoria, inappropriate laughter, and/or singing.

Similar anchor points are described for a total of eleven different symptoms. Some symptoms like aggressive or assaultive behavior are given more weight by rating the worst category as a 6 or an 8 instead of a 4. This is done because some symptoms are presumed to be more important than others in assessing the severity of the diagnosis. The total score is the total of the ratings on all eleven items and indicates the overall severity of the disorder.

The entire interview results are based on either the clinician's own observations or the oral self-report of the patient in response to questions. No attempt may be made to ascertain the time course of the various symptoms, their pervasiveness, or the current social context of the patient. If the patient exhibits very fast speech in the interview, for instance, the symptom could conceivably be present because the patient is in a big hurry to leave on that particular day but characterologically likes to make sure the doctor gets a very precise answer with all its myriad details to any question. The test assumes that the diagnosis has already been made using a complete diagnostic interview and that the diagnosis is correct.

If an office physician instead uses this checklist as a self-report instrument and bases the patient's initial evaluation primarily on it, then a significant risk is created for misdiagnosing a normal but perhaps maladaptive part of a person's personality as a symptom of another psychiatric disorder. Nowhere is this a bigger problem than for the diagnosis of bipolar disorder.

BIPOLAR DISORDER M.A.

Bipolar disorder, which was called manic-depressive illness forever prior to the name change in 1980, is not a subtle disorder. It is a disorder of mood characterized by periods of severe depression and other periods of extreme hyperactivity, with periods of *euthymia* (a range of normal mood states) in between. Persons in a manic state act in ways that are completely out of character for them, doing things that they themselves label crazy after they regain their senses, such as running up thousands of dollars on a credit card buying things they do not even need, or cheating on a spouse with a series of strange men picked up at bars they do not normally frequent. They are often psychotic—thinking, for example, that they have doctorate degrees in subjects they have never studied. A patient in a true manic state is hard to miss.

Many patients in a manic state are euphoric, but this is not necessarily the case. Sometimes they are more irritable than euphoric. This may be a case of what is informally called *dysphoric mania,* in which many manic symptoms are present but the patient nonetheless feels miserable. It is called a *mixed state* in the DSM, and is often misdiagnosed in patients who are not bipolar at all but merely emotionally unstable. In its true form, mixed states are again nearly unmistakable. Individuals who are just emotionally unstable are also today misdiagnosed as something called *bipolar II disorder.*

When manic patients become psychotic, they can develop symptoms that are identical to those seen in patients experiencing an acute exacerbation of schizophrenia. The doctor must determine the chronological course of the patient's symptoms in order to distinguish the two, and that has not always been done. In Chapter Six, I described the horrible consequences that can ensue when this error is made. When I was in training back in the mid-1970s, we were told that for every diagnosis made of acute mania in the United States, there were three diagnoses made of acute schizophrenia. In Great Britain, the numbers were exactly reversed. In the United States, mania was woefully underdiagnosed and schizophrenia overdiagnosed, particularly in African American patients.

The "experts" who talk about mania today maintain that is still underdiagnosed. In some hospital emergency rooms across the country confronted with acutely psychotic individuals, it may still be. However, outside of that setting, it is now overdiagnosed, and not just occasionally.

The label is being applied almost indiscriminately to any moody individual, most of whom have never been psychotic. In one study that was done using very careful diagnostic techniques,[2] nearly 40 percent of patients diagnosed with borderline personality disorder, the subject of the next chapter, were found to have been previously misdiagnosed with bipolar disorder. Slightly more than 10 percent of all the other patients in the study also had carried the misdiagnosis.

Manic-depressive illness has been described in many different cultures for literally hundreds of years, as have many other psychiatric disorders. If a new psychiatric disorder suddenly appears on the scene, this most likely means one of four things. The first way that "new" psychiatric disorders appear is the theme of this book. Normal reactions and behavior, as well as their neurophysiologic underpinnings and their aftermath, are turned into mental disorders. The other three ways are the following: the disorder was not known to doctors because the individuals who had it seldom came to medical attention; the disorder is due to the appearance of a new toxin or a new germ that has recently mutated, such as HIV; or the disorder's roots lie in cultural changes and the disorder is therefore psychological rather than strictly biogenetic in origin. Our genetic makeup has not suddenly changed in just a few decades in ways that would produce some new disease.

For decades, psychiatry residents were taught that the incidence of manic-depressive illnesses was about 1 percent of the population, about the same as schizophrenia. Now we hear figures as high as 4.4 percent, although this figure is said to include "subthreshold" cases.[3] The percentage of bipolar patients who responded to the wonder drug for this disorder, lithium, was thought earlier to be around 80 percent. This has now been revised downward to as little as 40 percent. What is going on here? Was organized psychiatry wrong all those years?

I do not think so. I believe that the incidence figures have gone up because the criteria being used by researchers have become more elastic. The rise in the incidence of bipolar disorder diagnoses has paralleled the rise in the concepts of *bipolar II disorder* and *bipolar spectrum disorder*. Bipolar II is supposedly a disorder in which affected individuals have severe depressive episodes but only very mild manic episodes called *hypomania*. Before looking critically at the bipolar II concept, I will first address reasons for the dwindling numbers that are quoted as the percentage of bipolar patients who respond to lithium.

Lithium

The experts who advocated for the inclusion of bipolar II in the DSM admit that patients who have it do not generally respond to lithium. Ipso facto, if such patients are included in studies, the percentage of subjects who are lithium responders goes down. Many patient samples in today's studies include patients diagnosed with both bipolar I and bipolar II. However, this is not the only reason why the lithium numbers have changed. I have seen researchers employ several sneaky tricks to make it appear that lithium is less effective than once thought.

Why is this done? I do not know for certain, but once again many of the newer drugs advertised as "mood stabilizers" are expensive brand-name medications, while lithium is a cheap generic. Lithium is not even really a drug; it is a salt. Its side effects are usually not serious in most patients, but a lot of doctors seem to think it has a lot of really bad side effects. Once again, the more the companies that make brand-name drugs expand the definition of mania and the more they discount the use of cheaper generic drugs, the more money they make. Unfortunately, the more this happens, the more that psychotherapy addressing what may be the real behavior problem is underutilized.

Interestingly, now that one of the other main drugs proven effective in treating true mania, Depakote, has lost its patent, we are suddenly hearing a lot more about the use in bipolar disorder of brand-name "atypical" antipsychotic medications, as well as a drug called Lamictal. We old-timers have always known that *all* antipsychotic medications, including the oldest, now generic ones, are effective in mania. Manufacturers of the old antipsychotics, available since the 1950s, never did studies on them for that indication, so the FDA never approved them for that use.

Getting back to the tricks used to discount lithium, in order to understand them, two characteristics of lithium must be appreciated. First, it is far more effective for both the acute treatment of a current episode and for the prevention of later episodes of bipolar mania than it is for bipolar depression. Second, it only works if the patient's blood level of the drug is high enough. Blood levels in patients taking lithium are supposed to be monitored closely, because the effective blood level is very close to the toxic blood level. Lithium toxicity can cause death, but the use of lithium in suicide attempts is rather low. This may be because it has, unlike other so-called mood stabilizers, an antisuicide effect, which is another reason it should be the first drug of choice for bipolar disorder.

Newer studies of lithium tend to look at its effectiveness for the prevention of future episodes of either mania *or* depression. If you combine all mood episodes instead of looking at just mania, this again naturally decreases the percentage of patients for whom it "works." Another trick is to include in the definition of "nonresponders" to the medication those who did not respond only because they were actually non-*compliant*. To point out the painfully obvious, if you do not take a medication, it does not tend to work all that well. If you do not take it as prescribed, and therefore have too low a level, it also will not work. If a published report of a study does not indicate that the subjects had frequently monitored lithium blood levels, it may be inflating the number of actual nonresponders for this reason.

When it became clear that two anticonvulsants, Depakote and Tegretol, were effective for the prophylaxis or prevention of mania in bipolar patients, the manufacturers of many other brand-name anticonvulsants got in the act. They were not allowed by the FDA, supposedly, to tout their drugs for indications like bipolar disorder that had not been FDA approved, but somehow word got out that a variety of anticonvulsants might be effective in bipolar disorders.

In contradistinction to the rules for pharmaceutical companies, once a drug is approved for one purpose by the FDA, doctors are free to prescribe it for anything they choose. Suddenly anticonvulsants like Neurontin were being widely used for allegedly bipolar patients by high numbers of psychiatrists. According to Angell,[4] the manufacturers of Neurontin actually got into hot water because they were touting it for a wide variety of other unapproved uses, such as for insomnia, hot flashes, and migraine headaches. They accomplished this mostly by paying academic experts to put their names on flimsy research and then disseminating the articles to doctors. In May 2004, the manufacturer of Neurontin was fined $430 million to resolve criminal charges and civil liabilities in connection with this deception. Later studies actually showed clearly than Neurontin was ineffective in bipolar disorder.

If a pharmaceutical company wants its drug for bipolar disorder to look really good, it can design studies using an outcome measure called *time to the next affective episode*, and compare it to placebo, not lithium. This outcome measure seems to have become somewhat of a fad after it was widely used in studies of Lamictal. When psychiatrists first heard about that drug, it was touted as the first drug that was specifically effective for bipolar depression. Somewhat surprisingly, when it received FDA approval, it was approved for bipolar disorder in general. Later studies showed that it was ineffective against an acute episode of bipolar depression, but that it might still be useful for prophylaxis of later episodes of bipolar depression. The studies on which the FDA based its initial approval of the drug used the questionable outcome measure.

If taken religiously and with the right blood levels, lithium truly prevents recurrences of mania. Lamictal was given to a number of supposedly well-diagnosed and stable or euthymic bipolar patients and the patients were monitored for eighteen months for the reemergence of either depressive or manic symptoms. The time that it took for each patient to experience a recurrence of any mood episode was measured and averaged, and using this yardstick, Lamictal beat placebo. Those taking Lamictal took longer, on the average, to have a recurrence of either mania or depression than those on placebo.

The trick here is that if a drug were truly prophylactic, then the compliant patient would *never* have another episode. Say the drug prevented recurrent episodes in just 2 or 3 percent of patients in the study for the full eighteen months. This would cause the average time to the next episode for the whole sample to go up, and the difference might easily be statistically but not clinically significant. Despite working for a few patients, the number of people for whom the drug was effective would be minimal. Even then, we would still not know if the drug was truly prophylactic for the people in the study who responded, because a significant number of patients with bipolar disorder have recurrences much less frequently than once every eighteen months.

Bipolar II Disorder

Unlike most major psychiatric diagnoses that have been known throughout much of history, bipolar II was nowhere to be found in the first two editions of the DSM. As residents in the mid-1970s we never heard about it, and, looking back, we never saw patients who might now "qualify" for the diagnosis by exhibiting the necessary signs and symptoms. It was first mentioned in the DSM III in 1980, but still was not listed as an official disorder. It was mentioned in the text that described a wastebasket diagnostic category called "atypical" bipolar disorder, which later morphed into "bipolar disorder not otherwise specified (NOS)" in the DSM III-Revised Edition in 1987. The atypical and NOS categories were reserved for patients who seemed to have some symptoms of a disorder in question, but not enough of them or of enough severity or duration to qualify for the official diagnosis.

Not until the DSM IV came out in 1994 did bipolar II receive enough support from the groups writing the DSM to become an official diagnosis. Hence, it appears that it took the powers that be at least fourteen years to decide clearly that this supposedly common disorder really exists. According to the DSM IV, the disorder occurs in 1 of every 200 people in the general population. By 1994, a virtual cottage industry of bipolar II research had sprung up.

In January 2009, drug company involvement in this explosion of new bipolar disorder diagnoses was clearly demonstrated by smoking-gun company memos that leaked out as part of a Justice Department settlement against the maker of the atypical antipsychotic Zyprexa for off-label marketing of the drug. These memos were supposed to be kept secret, but they were obtained by reporter Alex Berenson of the *New York Times*, as mentioned in an article in the paper on December 18, 2006. They were later put on the Internet by another reporter, Philip Dawdy of the *Seattle Weekly*, on his Furious Sessions Web site.

The memos indicate that a concerted effort was made to convince doctors, particularly those in family or internal medicine, that their patients with both anxiety and depression or impulse control problems might actually have bipolar disorder. The company succeeded in this endeavor beyond its wildest dreams, and a lot of psychiatrists came along for the ride.

Hypomania, one of the hallmarks of bipolar II, is characterized by mildly inflated self-esteem, grandiosity, decreased need for sleep, talkativeness, racing thoughts, distractibility, increased activity, and excessive involvement in potentially dangerous pleasurable activities. Hypomania is the only psychiatric syndrome in the DSM that does not require its sufferers to exhibit any distress or functional impairment. In fact, because an elevated mood is a major part of the syndrome, some people do really well when in that state. In bipolar disorder as it was originally conceptualized, hypomania was usually a prelude to a full-blown manic episode.

Since all of us experience symptoms of an elevated mood at one time or another, the writers of the DSM specified that hypomania must be clearly different from the patient's usual mood and behavior when in the euthymic state. In fact, it must be an unequivocal change in functioning that is uncharacteristic of the person when he or she is not symptomatic. This of course implies that there should be periods when the patient is asymptomatic or euthymic. Furthermore, the symptoms should last for more than just a few hours. The DSM committee responsible for the diagnostic criteria, in order to prevent normal everyday mood swings from being mislabeled, set the minimum duration for a hypomanic episode at four days. Admittedly this was an arbitrary number. Why not three days, or five?

If the intent of the DSM committee was to stop normal mood changes from being mislabeled by including these caveats, they failed miserably. Many clinicians, especially psychiatrists, began using the symptom checklists and context-avoiding diagnostic techniques previously described and began finding patients with the diagnosis under every tree.

Mania is one of most difficult psychiatric syndromes to describe to patients during diagnostic interviews. I find I often have to ask a question about manic symptoms in two or three different ways before patients clearly understand that I am asking about symptoms that are far above and beyond their usual experiences with mood changes, and that in a hypomanic or manic state they would act in ways that are totally out of character for them. The residents whom I observe doing diagnostic interviews all have the same problem. To think that a psychiatrist can accurately evaluate reports from patients about hypomanic or even manic symptoms using only a symptom checklist is ludicrous.

A Valid and Generalizable Anecdote

To illustrate this point, I will describe how this problem was manifested in a videotape that was sold to help psychiatry residents pass the oral examination from the American Board of Psychiatry and Neurology (ABPN) that allows them to call themselves board-certified psychiatrists. In the actual test, a real patient that is unknown to the examinee and two examiners comes for a half-hour diagnostic interview performed by the examinee. After the interview, examinees present the case and a treatment plan, and the examiners question them on anything the examinees bring up. This test is very difficult and has a very high failure rate. In fact, the ABPN is eliminating this part of the exam partially for this reason, but also for reasons of cost. As I have previously mentioned, it is impossible to obtain all of the information necessary to make an informed diagnosis in 30 minutes. The test is designed to allow an examinee to demonstrate an ability to prioritize and to think quickly on his or her feet.

Some otherwise excellent training videotapes, called *Pass the Boards*, were produced to demonstrate to residents potential pitfalls in taking the exam. They used real patients, real psychiatric residents, and real examiners to simulate the actual conditions of the board exam.

The patient in one particular videotape was described on the cover as having "features of bipolar disorder, rapid cycling, borderline personality disorder, and alcohol abuse." In the tape, the patient stated that she had recently been discharged from the hospital after being admitted for a medication adjustment. Over a period of years, she said she had been prescribed a wide variety of different psychiatric medications from different classes of drugs, none of which had been very helpful. She complained of mood swings. When asked how many days out of the year she had swings, she replied, "364." She also said during a different portion of the interview that she was depressed every day. The resident tried in vain to clarify if the patient ever had at any time during her life episodes in which all the symptoms of a clinical major depression were present at the same time.

The patient described one episode that sounded like it might have qualified. During this time in her life, she said she had spent a whole summer on the couch. She just could not get up at all. Later she mentioned, however, that during this same period she took her kids to the bus stop every morning and went to work almost every day, only calling in sick a handful of times. She also mentioned that during her depressed periods she could not sleep all night on numerous occasions. Insomnia is a symptom of a clinical depression. However, she added that she slept all day the next day. In watching the tape, I did not think the resident even heard that last part of her answer. Getting one's days and nights reversed is not insomnia at all.

The patient was asked about her "highs." She stated that her "highs" were never euphoric. She felt irritable, overwhelmed, and "hyper," yelled at her kids, and felt that unspecified family members were making her life miserable. She also said she really was not sure if she should be separating her highs from her lows, because when she was depressed, which as mentioned was pretty much all the time, she was also irritable.

Now of course I had the advantage, unlike the doctors in the videotape, of being able to watch the interview more than once, and to slow it down if necessary. One had to listen to the tape very carefully to understand what the patient was actually describing. From what I heard, she sounded to me like she was saying that when she was busy at work, she was not thinking about how bad she felt. When she got home she started to think more about her life, and began to feel bad. The bad feeling could be depression, irritability, or a mixture of both, depending on how her kids and the rest of her family were acting. She would then medicate her bad feelings with alcohol.

She alluded in the tape to many family-of-origin problems. She spoke of having revenge fantasies of someone hurting her adoptive mother, with whom she was usually angry. She said that in the past she had long fantasized about her biological mother, whom she had idealized until she had actually met the woman a few years before the interview was taped. The patient then found out that her biological mother could barely take care of herself, let alone the patient. The patient's depression got worse immediately following that meeting. The patient also mentioned almost in passing that she had been molested by a relative.

The examinee clearly did not think it a priority to ask for more details about these highly suggestive little tidbits about the patient's family life, even when she had a couple of minutes at the end of the interview that she could have used for that purpose. To their credit, the examiners later gave the resident the feedback that she should have devoted a little more of the interview to the social history, so as to rule out past trauma that might be associated with the unstable moods characteristic of borderline personality disorder, the subject of the next chapter.

They said they suspected that a trauma history was likely. Apparently every doctor in the room had either missed or forgotten about the patient's mention of the molestation. Part of being a good diagnostician is to listen very carefully for hints, often mentioned by a patient quickly and in hushed tones buried in discourse about unrelated topics, that might lead the examiner to a conclusion different from a more seemingly obvious one. Mental health professionals may seem to be "just listening," but the good ones really are concentrating and thinking. The poor resident could be excused for missing the statement about the molestation because she was nervous in the exam situation, but what about the two examiners?

During the time the examiners were questioning the resident, I heard one of them say, "This patient did describe quite clearly distinct times" during the day during which she felt quite different from other times. Clearly? Distinct? Although the patient was trying very hard to answer the interviewer's questions accurately and to please the doctor, she had hemmed, hawed, and then flat out contradicted herself when questioned about whether the lows and the hyper periods were actually distinct. Being unhappier in one's home environment than one is at work, or vice versa, is a sign that there may be a problem in one of the two environments. A mood swing that occurs when one goes from one to the other hardly qualifies for the diagnosis of bipolar disorder.

Even more astonishing than the examiner's statement about the clarity of the patient's descriptions of distinct mood periods was that both examiners seemed to agree with the resident when she made the primary diagnosis of bipolar disorder. If this resident is representative of how a lot of psychiatry residents are being trained nowadays, and I think it is, then I despair for the profession, not to mention for the patients saddled with stigmatizing diagnoses and then placed on unnecessary medications with serious side effects.

This patient's symptoms very clearly did not meet the DSM duration requirement for bipolar episodes. The *Pass the Board* tapes were made back in 1995, but if anything the problem of ignoring duration standards has become much worse since then. That clinical psychiatrists routinely ignore them in their diagnostic interviews is further illustrated by statements made frequently to me by my patients to the effect that "I was really manic last night."

Oh no, they were not. These patients were plainly not in anything approaching a manic state during my interview the very next day when they were saying this. Mania does not go away overnight. I even saw a patient on a videotaped psychotherapy session, who was becoming very agitated while discussing a very painful emotional experience, say, "Look at how manic I'm getting." I do not know for sure, but I assume these patients learned to use the term *manic* inappropriately from mental health practitioners who had treated them in the past.

From the start, the aforementioned cottage industry of researchers in so-called bipolar disorder were very unhappy about the duration criteria for bipolar II disorder specified in the DSM, and began to advocate for the position that a hypomanic episode could last any amount of time, no matter how short. In fact, they also believed that full-blown manic episodes did not have to last the DSM mandated seven days, particularly as previously mentioned, in children.

Many of them began to talk about bipolar disorder as existing on a wide "spectrum." They even talked about bipolar III or even bipolar IV disorder, or, as I used to joke with the residents, bipolar version 2.1. I guess if an individual wins the lottery and stays up all night partying in a state of euphoria, he or she must be bipolar. Since spending sprees may be a symptom of mania, anyone who runs up charges on a credit card is at risk of being labeled as having a manic symptom. Of course, when psychiatrists do this, they disregard the fact that an incredibly high percentage of the population of the United States has amassed significant credit card debt.

Many of my patients with trauma histories, personality disorders, and chaotic families were misdiagnosed as bipolar with absolutely no symptoms suggestive of the true disorder at all. I began to refer to phony bipolar diagnoses as "bipolar m.a."—bipolar, my ass. Nowhere is this insanity more outrageous than in the current rush to diagnose very young, acting-out children, not as ADHD, but as bipolar.

Bipolar Disorder in Children

In the last few years, a Harvard psychiatrist named Joseph Biederman began to gain a lot of traction and influence in the psychiatric profession with studies that purported to show that bipolar disorder could be diagnosed in children as young as three. His previous area of interest was, not surprisingly, ADHD, a subject on which I also have a very different opinion.

The fact that Biederman is a psychiatrist from Harvard, one of the most prestigious and highly rated medical schools, and has published a large number of papers bolstered his claims. However, his methods for diagnosing bipolar disorder in children were highly unsatisfactory to my mind, at least according to the way they were described in his publications. He mostly reported basing diagnoses purely on symptom reports by parents and teachers. His articles rarely report *any* significant evaluation of the psychosocial context in which the symptoms of his subjects took place, an evaluation that might suggest that the subjects' problem was agitation or acting out, not mania.

I have no direct knowledge about how good a scientist Dr. Biederman actually is or how carefully he screens his study subjects, and I am not accusing him of anything. I do know, however, that Dr. Biederman got into some hot water. A *New York Times* report dated June 8, 2008, reported about Biederman, "A world-renowned Harvard child psychiatrist whose work has helped fuel an explosion in the use of powerful antipsychotic medicines in children earned at least $1.6 million in consulting fees from drug makers from 2000 to 2007 but for years did not report much of this income to university officials, according to information given Congressional investigators." The fact that he did not disclose this obvious conflict of interest is troublesome.

As I have already mentioned, whenever the topic of diagnosing bipolar disorder in young children comes up in throwaway journals,

I seem to see the mantra that bipolar symptoms in children probably do not have to meet DSM duration criteria. In fact, these kids are said to have several mood swings *in one day.* This is often said as if it is an established fact whose validity has been accepted by the entire profession. The people who say this are just making up their own absurd criteria out of thin air because they do not like the ones in the DSM. No widely accepted science of any sort supports this idea. Any biological "abnormalities" they quote, as we have seen in Chapter Four, prove nothing of the sort.

Of interest is the frequent report by the advocates for diagnosing bipolar disorder in young children that the illness in kids does not generally respond to lithium treatment. The usual explanation is that pediatric bipolar disorder is "different" than it is in adults. Could it be that the reason that pediatric bipolar disorder does not respond to lithium is that these children are not bipolar in the first place? So which drugs do these experts usually recommend? Those old familiar expensive brand-name atypical antipsychotic drugs that seem to be good for whatever else ails you. Most of these drugs had never been tested in pediatric populations at the time of this writing.

Since the alleged symptoms of mania in children look suspiciously similar to acting out, one wonders how a psychiatrist who does not even look at family behavior can really tell the difference. The symptoms also look a lot like the symptoms of ADHD. In fact, many children have been diagnosed with both bipolar disorder *and* ADHD, and they are prescribed both a stimulant and a central nervous system depressant, many of whose effects cancel each other out from a pharmacological point of view. The same children often carry still other additional diagnoses that all smack of acting-out behavior: *oppositional defiant disorder* and *conduct disorder.* These are behavior problems that used to be called juvenile delinquency.

I should acknowledge that it is indeed true that if one of the parents of a hyperactive or any other type of child has true bipolar disorder, the child is at fairly high risk of developing the disorder later in life. Estimates are that about 10 percent of the children who have one parent with bipolar disorder will develop the disease at some point. The risk is higher than that if other closely related individuals have it. The question is, however, whether the hyperactive behavior of such a child is due to an early manifestation of the disorder or if it is just plain acting out due to inconsistent and/or abusive discipline. I frankly do not see how a clinician can tell, especially if the family dynamics are superficially evaluated. A second question is, even if the behavior is an early manifestation of the disorder, should it be treated with potentially toxic drugs that might cause diabetes in some of the children? Might not family intervention with psychotherapy stop the problem behavior more safely?

John Rosemond has a book called *The Diseasing of America's Children* that covers some of the same territory I am covering in this chapter. He believes the change during the last forty years in the predominant parenting style, as I have previously discussed, is by far the biggest reason for unruly behavior in children. Indirect evidence that kids from bad environments are being mislabeled with biogenetic disorders is the fact that children in foster care in Texas are given heavy psychiatric medicines at a rate far greater than that seen for children not in foster care.[5] No reason exists to think that children in foster care have more genetic liability for bipolar disorder than other children, but foster children often come from a high-risk environment.

Drugs, Anyone?

The absurd lengths to which some psychiatrists go to diagnose bipolar disorder and, as we shall see, adult ADHD is known among some frequent-flyers on psychiatric inpatient units. They sometimes even laugh about it behind the backs of the doctors and nurses, and trade stories about how they fool everybody. As a psychiatrist myself, I of course do not usually hear these stories directly, but the occasional honest patient tells me or my resident about them. My favorite story came from one patient who had herself been diagnosed as bipolar. She knew very well that her problems and symptoms had instead been created because she had come from a dysfunctional and chaotic family of origin, with whom she still had to deal on a daily basis. She spoke of one hospital inpatient unit in Memphis notorious for doctors who strained at making dubious diagnoses. She said, "There was a lot of diagnonsense going on around there." Out of the mouths of babes . . .

I did not ask her about it, but undoubtedly many of the young patients on her ward also knew that if they just complained about the right symptoms, their psychiatrists might prescribe stimulants for them. This occurs not only in psychiatric hospitals, but in psychiatrists' offices as well. If these patients were to instead ask for benzodiazepines, which are much safer drugs, they would immediately arouse suspicion that they were "drug seekers." As we have seen, benzos are less expensive than the new longer-acting brand-name stimulants, and drug companies have a financial interest in grossly exaggerating their dangers and abuse potential.

Psychiatrists need to face the fact that the symptoms of many psychiatric disorders are easy to fake. In children, parents are not beyond coaching their kids to fake psychiatric disorders for financial gain. This is illustrated by a fairly well-known scam known as *crazy checks*, in which parents coach their children to act crazy to qualify them for Social Security Disability. Crazy checks usually go to people already receiving other public assistance checks who have become adept at milking the system for more.

ADULT ADHD: ANOTHER DUBIOUS HYPED DISORDER

I was recently asked by my department to help out a couple of hours per week seeing patients at the University Student Mental Health Service. Our university campus has no undergraduate students; all of the students are professional school attendees such as medical, dental, nursing, and pharmacist students, as well as master's and PhD students in the health sciences. I did not see any printed statistics from the service, but I was told by the psychiatrist in charge that approximately one-fourth of the students who consulted the Student Mental Health Service were taking stimulants for "adult attention deficit disorder," mostly the "inattentive" rather than the "hyperactive" subtype.

Some of these students had been taking these medications since grade school, but a lot of them had not been previously diagnosed with the childhood version of the disorder. The DSM requires that symptoms of ADHD must have been present since at least the age of seven in order to make the diagnosis, because all of the so-called science behind the diagnosis indicates that it never begins in adolescence or adulthood.

The fact that so many of our students were being diagnosed in adulthood struck me as particularly odd since these students, who supposedly had trouble concentrating in class, had been able to do so well in high school and college that they had managed to get admitted into extremely competitive academic programs. For many of them, nearly straight A grades had been required. If these students were unable to concentrate, one would shudder to think what they might have been able to accomplish if they could.

A psychologist on our faculty who evaluates the students in our school who come to the Student Mental Health Center complaining of ADHD-like symptoms compared a sample of them to a sample of students who were not seeking treatment. Interestingly, almost as high a percentage of students in the group that was not seeking help seemed to meet criteria for the ADHD diagnosis as in the group of students who were.

Speed

I was horrified to learn of the extent of on-campus amphetamine and Ritalin use and let the service know not to refer me any patients who were seeking those drugs. I almost never prescribe them. The dangers of stimulants are significant, and the benefits are questionable. The drugs do help calm hyperactive children down over the short term, but their long-term benefits for improving social and occupational functioning in these children are at best minimal.

Everyone knows about how bad cocaine is, and cocaine is also a stimulant that does many of the same things as Ritalin and amphetamines. The drugs can cause cardiac problems, such as those that killed the twenty-two-year-old basketball player Len Bias in 1986. They can cause psychosis. They are often abused, even when prescribed by a physician. In the 1950s and 1960s, amphetamines were routinely prescribed to housewives as diet pills. Many of these women became strung out. Doctors eventually stopped prescribing them for weight loss because amphetamines deservedly developed a bad reputation. The singer Johnny Cash was famously known for his erratic behavior when he was using them.

I remembered what the hippies in the Haight Ashbury district used to say about them during my freshman year at Berkeley in 1966 and 1967. They used to say "speed kills," and they were not talking about driving too fast. That particular sentiment came from people who were *in favor* of getting high on a variety of other drugs!

Furthermore, I read in the newspaper that an epidemic was breaking out on college campuses of students using the drugs to get ahead of the competition for positions in postgraduate schools. The drugs not only help people who have been diagnosed with ADHD concentrate. They help almost anyone concentrate much better. People can take them and study all night. On campuses across the country, they are nicknamed *academic steroids*, because they are in fact performance-enhancing drugs, only for intellectual rather than for athletic performance. If athletes who take steroids are cheating, then so are students who take amphetamines. Cheating in school, as evidenced by such activities as plagiarizing papers off the Internet, has unfortunately become almost acceptable among college students.

Some of the students who use "academic steroids" use stashes of drugs taken from younger siblings who are taking them for the diagnosis of ADHD. Just as an aside, this may run somewhat counter to studies that purport to show that children who take stimulants for ADHD are no more prone to abuse or divert drugs for profit when they get older than are those who do not take them. Perhaps the authors of these studies should have looked at these kids' older siblings. Of course, a lot of the older students are getting them directly from doctors. Lately, obtaining them from legitimate physicians has not been all that difficult.

Journals and psychiatric newspapers have recently been inundated with advertisements for stimulants. One, Adderall XR, is a long-acting drug that contains as an ingredient the old diet medicine Dexedrine. Its effects are not all that different from those of methamphetamine, the abuse of which is considered a national emergency. Along with the ads are helpful articles about how to treat adults with the disorder. For example, an article entitled "ADHD in Adults: Matching Therapies with Patients' Needs" appeared in the journal *Current Psychiatry* dated September 2008.[6] This journal advertises itself as evidence-based and peer-reviewed.

As a diagnostic aid, the article recommends that clinicians employ a self-report symptom checklist called the World Health Organization Adult ADHD Self Report Scale. The fact that this instrument appears to be endorsed by the World Health Organization makes it sound very impressive indeed. Some of the items on the checklist include: "How often do you have difficulty getting things in order when you have to do a task that requires organization?" "When you have a task that requires a lot of thought, how often do you avoid or delay getting started?" "How often do you fidget or squirm with your hands or feet when you have to sit down for a long time?"

My goodness! I almost always fidget with my foot when I have to sit through long lectures. Maybe I have ADHD. It seems more likely that some very common behavioral problems such as being disorganized and procrastinating have suddenly and magically been turned into symptoms of a mental disorder. The authors of this particular article go on to mention that symptoms of ADHD often fluctuate over time. How convenient.

The article describes the case of a man who had ADHD symptoms and who, they mention in passing, was intermittently subject to "minor" depression, whatever that is. He was having trouble at his job after a promotion led to a significant increase in his workload. Could it be that this man was merely unhappy with his job, or felt overworked and overwhelmed? The authors do say that he had a history of these symptoms when he was in high school and college. Does that exclude the current job as a source of his symptoms? That seems to be what the article implies. Of course, he may have been unhappy with other aspects of his life back then, but no matter.

The kicker was a sentence on page 56 of the article that said, in regards to his academic performance, that the man "just got by . . . by cramming in high school and college." *Cramming?* I always thought cramming meant sitting for a relatively extended period of time and pushing as much information into one's head as possible. I thought having ADHD meant that he would not have been able to do that.

The authors of the article go on to assure readers that, at least in children, use of stimulants does not lead to increased risk for later substance abuse. The reference for this is an article by . . . Joseph Biederman. This conclusion was reached despite studies that show that prescribed stimulants are often diverted by college students to nonmedical uses[7] and that calls made to poison control centers regarding stimulant abuse rose 76 percent from 1998 to 2005.[8]

ADHD IN CHILDREN

As many readers are aware, many professionals and laypeople alike, and not just Scientologists, have long thought that the diagnosis of ADHD in children is made way too often. Some have questioned the legitimacy of the diagnosis entirely. Over the years parents have sometimes been pressured by schoolteachers to put their kids on stimulants just to quiet them down. In this section, I do not mean to sound like Tom Cruise: someone who attacks the profession (to which I myself belong) to advance the insane Scientology agenda. But, as they say, even a broken cuckoo clock is right twice a day, especially when the facts unfortunately lend support to its position.

The DSM symptoms of the *inattentive* form of the disorder are "often" making careless mistakes on schoolwork, having trouble paying attention and listening when spoken to, not finishing assignments or chores, trouble organizing and making a mental effort, losing things needed for tasks and activities, and being easily distracted. The symptoms of the *hyperactive-impulsive* type are "often" fidgeting, getting up from their seats when they should not, running or climbing inappropriately, having trouble playing quietly, acting as if on the go, talking excessively, blurting out answers to questions, trouble waiting one's turn, and interrupting and intruding upon others.

"Often" is not defined precisely. The criteria of not following instructions and failing to finish work assignments, the DSM says, must not be due to "oppositional behavior." How one can tell for certain whether or not a child who is not following instructions or finishing homework is being oppositional, one can only guess.

All of these characteristics are shown by almost all children naturally at one time or another. If they have a lot of them frequently, their behavior may be due to their being chronically anxious or upset. Such kids have trouble sitting still. Children who come from families with highly inconsistent and/or frankly abusive discipline can and often do show all of these symptoms much of the time. Acting out is a phenomenon well known to psychoanalysts and family therapists alike.

I am not a child psychiatrist, but my residents report that in our child and adolescent psychiatry clinic, which does assess the family environment, kids previously diagnosed with ADHD or pediatric bipolar disorder almost always seem to come from highly disturbed families. We may only be referred the most severely impaired cases, but I have no reason to think this is the case. One study[9] showed that children of parents in the midst of getting a divorce were almost twice as likely to be put on Ritalin as children whose parents were staying together. I wonder why that could be.

Sometimes a single clinical anecdote, although possibly valid for only that case, can be an exception that brings a rule into question. Actually, I have heard many clinical anecdotes that indicate that clear acting out or anxiety in children is easily and often confused with ADHD. In this example, a colleague discussed a child he had treated for ADHD who had all the symptoms of the disorder. The problem behavior was pervasive, persistent, and prominent and led to significant school impairment. The child was treated with a stimulant and had an excellent response. He calmed down considerably. Then, the child and his mother disappeared for over a year from my colleague's practice. They then returned as suddenly as they had disappeared. The mother asked that the child again be put on the stimulant, because the child was showing all the same symptoms. The doctor asked what had happened during their absence from his clinic.

The mother said that she had moved out of state. Knowing the importance of follow-up questions, my colleague inquired about whether the child was treated with the medication by another doctor in the state she had moved to. She replied that the child had not needed to take any. He had been calm and doing quite well in school without medication the entire time they were away. The symptoms had only arisen again when they had moved back. On further questioning, the mother told a hair-raising story of their violent living situation in my colleague's town. She had left the bad situation when she moved, and returned to it when she moved back.

Note that the mother did not even tell the psychiatrist what was really going on in their home until confronted with two quick and drastic changes in the level of the child's symptoms. While the medication was helpful in this case, clearly the horrific environment in which this child found himself, one that would over time create for this child far more problems than just trouble sitting still, needed to be addressed. The fact that "biological" psychiatrists often have no time to even ask about environmental issues is troublesome.

To me this type of clinical anecdote shows, assuming that the child did indeed have all of the symptoms of ADHD, that one of three things must be true. First, the doctor may not have applied the appropriate diagnostic criteria. I have no reason to think so in this particular case. Second, perhaps no doctor can tell from symptoms alone if this behavior is due to an underlying disorder or is a reaction to a discordant family environment. The third possibility is that the underlying disorder itself is really a normal psychological reaction to a problematic environment.

I once read in a psychiatric newspaper that the symptoms of ADHD were indistinguishable from the behavior of children who are at the high end of the normal bell-shaped curve for innate activity level. The author advised that the following criteria be applied: Anyone who seemed to be in the top 5 percent on this curve should be considered to have ADHD. That is like saying that all players in the National Basketball Association should be diagnosed with the disease acromegaly, an excess production of growth hormone, because they are all so tall.

ADHD in the Natural Habitat

The television show *Supernanny*, which actually takes cameras into the homes of its subjects, seems to show that this untrained but nonetheless effective family therapist is able to change a set of parents' behavior in ways that lead to improvements in the behavior of their out-of-control children, just like a good animal trainer changes the behavior of a dog's owner rather than merely training the animal. When the Supernanny leaves the household after she helps the parents' behavior to change, the parents usually revert to their old habits, and their children again act up. She then comes back and works on the problem again, and the earlier improved behavior of the children returns.

I can already hear my critics protesting that *Supernanny* is a simplistic television show, not real family therapy, and that the director is picking and choosing which families to show, and that the families that are shown are atypical. The family may be hamming it up for the cameras. In a given family, the director is also picking which interactions to show the audience and which not to show. TV executives want the Supernanny to look good, so this selection is biased and presents an incorrect picture of what is really going on. We cannot even be sure that some of the scenes we witness are not scripted or set up by the television crew. Maybe the show is another case of lemmings being driven over a cliff.

All this could very well be true. All I can say with confidence is that the scenarios that are portrayed on this show are consistent with the descriptions of family life I hear time and again from my adult patients from dysfunctional families, or that I have at times personally witnessed in my interactions with friends and neighbors. As for my patients' stories, I will discuss the evidence I use to support my belief in their truthfulness in Chapter Eight. In *Supernanny*, the family is at least being observed in its native habitat. That's more than I can say about the families in studies of ADHD and bipolar disorder in children.

It is noteworthy that in most of the studies about children with ADHD, as with pediatric bipolar disorder, the family environment of the subjects is not critically evaluated. If it is assessed at all, the evaluation usually consists primarily of asking parents to report on their own behavior, as if abusive or guilt-ridden parents are going to tell the truth about that in a relatively short meeting with a complete stranger.

The Party Line

Those psychiatrists who believe in only the biological and genetic underpinnings of the diagnosis are aware of these study limitations, but many seem to have a misleading counterargument at the ready. In different settings with different psychiatrists, I have heard that psychosocial issues as a primary cause of ADHD have been ruled out in some studies. I wonder if that statement is another one of those ideas that have been repeated so often and in so many different venues that they have become a sort of party line. The more a lie is repeated, the more it is believed.

One of these incidents took place in an exchange of letters I had in the professional newspaper the *Psychiatric Times*. It started with a letter to the editor from a Dr. Stephen Pitelli about an article by Dr. Karen Wagner that had been previously published in the paper. Dr. Wagner's article described the results of one particular treatment study of ADHD in children. Dr. Pitelli expressed concern about the powerful drugs being used to treat ADHD in preschoolers while family and psychosocial issues are being ignored.

In the letter to the editor section of psychiatric newspapers, authors who are criticized in a letter usually get to respond before the letter is published, and the response is printed immediately following the letter. Unfortunately, they almost always get the last word, so they are able to get away with things that they would not be able to in other contexts.

Dr. Wagner replied that the drugs in the study she wrote about were used only in patients who continued to meet DSM criteria for ADHD after ten weeks of parent training. This statement sounded to me like she was saying that family dysfunction had been ruled out, that the parent training had in a sense controlled for this. I was impressed by how Dr. Wagner was so enamored by the effectiveness of a psychosocial intervention, and apparently believed that ten weeks of parenting education could completely reverse years of well-ingrained parental habits. In response, I sent in my own letter to the editor, which was published in the April 2008 issue.

I wrote that she seemed to be implying that inconsistent and/or abusive parenting, which is a well-observed cause of acting out in children, could be cured in ten weeks. For this to be true, the parents would have to have consistently and scrupulously adhered to a complex new behavior pattern after this short instruction period. I pointed out that compliance studies on how often people follow instructions show that a significant percentage of them frequently do not consistently do so. This applies to instructions as simple as taking a pill. I could have perhaps added to my letter that following instructions consistently may have been particularly difficult for these parents, whose main difficulty with their children may have been inconsistency.

Even if parents who had been using problematic parenting strategies for quite some time did somehow benefit from the brief training to the maximum degree, one would still expect them to revert occasionally to their old problematic style out of sheer force of habit. Under these circumstances, occasional parental lapses would affect the child's behavior adversely even more than if they continued to do the wrong thing all the time.

The reason for this is has to do with something learning theorists refer to as a *variable intermittent reinforcement schedule*. Habits like acting out that have been reinforced occasionally and unpredictably by repetitive parenting errors become even more ingrained than those reinforced regularly. If the parents suddenly change their parenting style for the better, children will try very hard indeed to get them to change it back by escalating acting out to levels that are even higher than before. This reinforcement schedule is the reason for the success of slot machines in casinos. Occasional payoffs lead patrons, despite their losses, to persist longer in pulling the lever than they would otherwise.

In Dr. Wagner's reply to my letter, she said that she had made no implication about inconsistent or abusive parenting. She invited readers to obtain the study in question to look at its design and methodology. So, was she saying that the study had no implications at all about probably the most important psychosocial risk factors? That was sort of the point of Dr. Pitelli's original letter. What did the parent training in the study address—*irrelevant* parenting practices? I felt Dr. Wagner had completely sidestepped my criticism.

Giving her the benefit of the doubt, I then thought that perhaps Dr. Wagner was merely saying that psychosocial issues were not completely ignored in the study. I took her up on her invitation and looked at the original journal article.[10] She was right. There was no mention specifically of inconsistent or abusive discipline. However, on page 1276 the article stated, quite unequivocally, "Parent training was added to screen out children whose disruptive behaviors were more attributable to problematic parent-child interactions." This was precisely what I had thought she was implying in her original response to Dr. Pitelli. If indeed Dr. Wagner was correct about what behavior patterns the parent training in the study had addressed, then the authors of the study had not even come close to ruling out problematic parent-child interactions in their sample.

Yet another example of spurious reasoning concerning whether ADHD children truly have an inability to concentrate is also another great example of how so-called experts can adopt a party line. I once heard an "expert" make the interesting statement that, when an ADHD child is in a video arcade and is able to focus intently on the game, with distracting buzzers, bells, and lights going off all over the place and throngs of other people walking about in different directions, that the child's focus on the game in this situation is not the same thing as "concentration." This explanation seems to be a staple of ADHD researchers. They have to find a way to explain away data that do not fit with their ideas.

Leaving aside the fact that children diagnosed with ADHD are often able to demonstrate concentration in a variety of other environmental contexts, if what the child is doing at the arcade is not "concentration," then what, pray tell, is it? Advocates for this point of view may say that concentration on video games is different from other forms of concentration because the flickering screen has hypnotic properties and the individual therefore goes into an altered mental state, but that is complete conjecture.

Different brain parts are involved in different activities during which concentration is maintained. If you are concentrating while reading a book, different parts of the brain will light up on a PET scan than when you are concentrating on an audiotape of the same material being read aloud. That does not prove that retaining one's focus is a completely different skill in these two cases, although an individual can be naturally better at it in one context than the other. What scientific evidence do individuals making the patently absurd assertion that the child in a video arcade is not concentrating have to back it up? I will tell you: there isn't any. They just *made it up*. Again, repeat a lie often enough, and it becomes accepted as the truth.

As for the use of stimulants in children, during a professional meeting I once heard a bizarre and astonishing statement made by a representative of NIDA, the National Institute for Drug Abuse. During his lecture, he spoke about some alarming new findings concerning the effects on drug users of stimulants from the street. New studies had indicated that the drugs deplete a neurochemical called dopamine in certain parts of the brain that are responsible for the normal experiences of being rewarded and of feeling pleasure. Because of this, users have to use more and more of the stimulant to get the same effect. (Actually, chronic cocaine abusers have often told me and other doctors I know that they no longer experience any high at all from the drug, but nonetheless they mysteriously keep taking it.) Furthermore, chronic users are no longer able to normally experience pleasure in other usually enjoyable activities such as eating and having sex.

For some reason, that night I did not feel like being my usual contrarian self and stepping to the microphone at the conclusion of his talk to ask the lecturer a question about this. Luckily, someone else came up and asked him the very question I had in mind. The questioner asked if we were not creating this problem in children who are prescribed stimulants for ADHD. The response of the lecturer was positively jaw dropping. I was not recording the lecture, so I do not have his answer on tape, but it had such a dramatic impact on me that I do not think I am misquoting him. He replied, "But the drugs work so well!"

Wow. Was this man somehow in the pockets of pharmaceutical companies? I do not know. He obviously completely sidestepped the question that he was asked. He was saying, in effect, that the consequences of taking street amphetamines were really, really bad, but exactly the same consequences caused by a pharmaceutical company amphetamine could be safely ignored.

Adult patients diagnosed with bipolar II or ADHD, at least the ones I have seen over many years in a variety of different clinical settings, usually turn out not to actually meet the DSM criteria. Most of them turn out to have personality disorders. Some biological psychiatrists think that personality disorders will also turn out to be biogenetic diseases. I believe it more likely that most of them are understandable reactions and volitional interpersonal behaviors that are adaptive to troubled environments. To look further at this debate, in the next chapter I will discuss what has been termed the personality disorder without a specialty, borderline personality disorder. The content of debates about how best to treat this disorder provides a telling example of the trend toward pathologizing problematic behavior that stems primarily from dysfunctional family interactions.

8

Spinning on Axis II: The Mystery of Borderline Personality Disorder

I began a solo private practice in psychiatry way back in 1979. As most other doctors did, I decided to share call with other solo practitioners in the area to cover nights and weekends when I would be unavailable to take urgent or emergency calls from my patients. The first week that I was on-call for the group, our answering service phoned me at about 10 P.M. on a Friday night. The operator had something of a chuckle in her voice, which gave me the impression that she was thinking, "Wait until you get a load of this one." I told the operator to put the call through. The conversation went something like this:

> *Me:* "Hi, I'm Dr. Allen. I'm covering for Dr. [so and so]. What's up?"
> *Female voice:* "Doctor, I need help."
> *Me:* "What seems to be the problem?" For a few seconds, a stony silence prevailed. Then:
> *Patient:* "I just told you. *I need help.*"
> *Me:* "Well, what's wrong?
> *Patient:* "How am I supposed to know? *You're* the doctor."
> *Me:* "Well, can you tell me a little about what you are experiencing?" Another stony silence of a few seconds occurred.
> *Patient:* "Doctors *do* help people, *don't they?*"
> *Me:* "Well of course. Tell me about what's happening."
> *Patient (shouting):* "Why don't you want to help me?"
> *Me:* "Do you need to change your medication?"
> *Patient (with irritation and sarcasm oozing out of every syllable):* "How is *that* going to help me?"

This conversation went on like that for nearly an hour. She gave me absolutely no information about what was really bothering her or what sort of help she was seeking, but nonetheless kept insisting that I provide it for her. She implied that I was purposefully and spitefully holding back a solution to her problem, whatever it was. Before the end of the conversation, the patient was threatening me with lawsuits and the outside possibility that she might at some point commit suicide.

Having never been trained to deal with this sort of behavior in my residency, I eventually just threw up my hands in frustration and told her she would have to talk to her regular doctor the next day, and then hung up. Only later did I learn that this particular patient had pulled the exact same routine with every other member of my call panel the first time each of them had taken call for the group. How nice of my colleagues to warn me. I heard a rumor that one of the other doctors had gotten so angry at this patient that he told her that she was a dog and that she should have consulted a veterinarian.

This patient was obviously not stupid. She *had to have known* that if she did not give me any information about what her problem was then in no way would I be able to help her. Of course, whatever her problems were, they were most likely to be chronic, complex, difficult to unravel, and would take months or years to treat in psychotherapy. Why on Earth would she call doctors new to the call schedule and go on like this?

Back then, the diagnosis that this patient would now carry, borderline personality disorder (BPD), was not listed in the DSM. It did not make its appearance in the DSM until the third addition in 1980. Psychiatrists, particularly psychoanalysts, had been talking about it before then, but it was thought to be relatively uncommon. Such patients were thought to be "on the borderline" between psychosis and neurosis.

Psychoanalysts used to believe that behavioral problems due to internal conflicts (neurosis) exist on a continuum with psychotic disorders, in that all such disorders were psychological in origin and not due to brain pathology. "Borderline" patients were thought to be on the border between neurosis and psychosis. The syndrome was also called by a variety of other names, such as "pseudoneurotic schizophrenia." Informally, psychiatrists would facetiously and pejoratively refer to these patients by less fancy names like "help-rejecting complainers." They were thought to be unanalyzable, meaning that they were poor candidates for psychoanalytic treatment.

For a long time, both before and after BPD was included in the DSM, patients who carried the diagnostic label were believed to have transient or short-lived psychotic episodes. In truth, they never really have the delusions or hallucinations that warrant such a label; what they sometimes do just *seems* so crazy. A five-foot woman who starts to beat on a six-foot policeman who is trying to arrest her should by all rights be insane. However, she is not psychotic if she knows that he is a policeman, not a Martian, and also knows that she will get the worse of the two of them in a scuffle. Patients with BPD who go into a rage just do not *care* about what will happen to them. In the last version of the DSM, edition four, this criterion for the disorder was correctly changed to transient paranoid ideation or dissociative symptoms (a dreamlike state) when a patient is under stress.

BORDERLINE RAGE

When patients diagnosed with BPD go into a rage, the appearance and frequency of which are one of the other current diagnostic criteria for the disorder, one can easily understand why they were labeled as psychotic. I had a firsthand look at such a storm while working at a hospital job I had taken just out of training. Lucky for me, the patient was a small female, or I would not be alive to write this today. She seemed to be doing well, and I told her she was going to be discharged from the hospital. When she objected, I rather curtly, sternly, and insensitively dictated to her that she had to leave.

In a nanosecond, she stopped being the docile patient she had been in the hospital up to that point and went into a blind and violent rage. Without warning, she grabbed the table lamp from my desk and smashed it, and then came right at me with its sharp point. Somehow I managed to grab it before I was stabbed and literally wrestled her to the floor. My office was out of hearing range from the ward nursing station, so I was on my own. She next reached up and grabbed the telephone off the desk—this was in the days when a telephone actually weighed enough to function as a blunt instrument—and tried to bash me over the head with it. Again I was able to wrestle it away from her, but it took quite an effort. Even small people can gather a lot of strength when the adrenaline is flowing. We finally rolled out the door into the hallway where the nurses could see us, and they pulled her off of me. All of this happened only because I told her I was going to discharge her from a mental hospital.

Who in their right mind wants or likes to stay in a mental hospital? No wonder people who acted like this were labeled psychotic. Of course, perhaps I should have asked her what was waiting for her at home, since she so dreaded returning there. Knowing nothing about the reasons behind her attack, I immediately ordered that she be whisked off to the nearest state mental hospital. I did not know what else to do. Strangely, just before she left she came up to me and sheepishly apologized for trying to kill me.

I had one other occasion to witness borderline rage that I will describe shortly. In that case the violence was thankfully not directed at me. Nonetheless, I never want to see it again. Later I learned that there are some simple ways to prevent it from arising in my office.

SELF-INJURIOUS BEHAVIOR

Another activity characteristic of patients with BPD is referred to as *self-injurious behavior* (SIB) or *deliberate self-harm.* Individuals with BPD cut themselves or burn themselves with cigarettes, usually without any intent to commit suicide, because for some reason they seem to feel better afterwards. They may also hit themselves or even, in very extreme and thankfully rare cases, do self-amputations of body parts. Some of us believe that the bulimic symptom of self-induced vomiting may also qualify as SIB. Multiple body piercing and tattoos may also represent SIB in some cases.

BPD patients do frequently threaten to commit suicide, make suicide gestures, or make actual attempts, but SIB per se is not necessarily connected with suicidality. When I was in training in the 1970s, patients who cut their wrists were assumed to be making suicide attempts. In my residency training we had heard almost nothing about nonpsychotic individuals who injured themselves on purpose without suicidal intent. I had not seen, nor even heard about, patients who burned themselves until I treated such a person during that hospital job I took right after my psychiatry residency.

WHO NEEDS THE AGGRAVATION?

In mental health circles, patients with BPD are generally most famous for being impossibly aggravating, although this attribute is not one of the diagnostic criteria. Sometimes difficult patients who do not meet criteria for BPD are labeled as borderlines just because they are difficult. I was able to build a practice in a region of the country that had many competing psychiatrists just by accepting referrals of these patients, as other therapists and psychiatrists could hardly wait to be rid of them. The referring clinicians used to apologize to me profusely for sending them to me.

To further illustrate what I mean by aggravating, I will describe another patient who exemplified this quality. In fact, she was the first patient I saw as a psychotherapist in training. After a couple of sessions, I was seriously questioning my sanity for having chosen a career as a therapist. The patient started our first session by literally doing nothing but insulting me for the entire hour, which she continued to do for several more sessions. She complained about everything from my inexperience, an obviously accurate assessment, to my looks.

She compared me to the resident whom I had replaced as her doctor. According to the patient, the prior resident was just perfect, except for the fact that she had abandoned the patient and left her in my care. Compared to the last therapist, she said, I was an unfeeling, incompetent little rodent. She then went to my primary supervisor to complain about me—an unnerving experience for any trainee. She told him I was ruining her. He, being very savvy, told her that he would not assign her to another resident. She was told that she should try to work things out with me first, because if she did, she would probably learn something about herself.

She came back to me and gradually settled down, and stopped the tirade of insults. Her treatment actually became quite productive. At the end of the year, when it was my turn to "abandon" her, she began to discuss her behavior at the beginning of the year. She was not speaking in retrospect, as though she had gained some new insight. She told me about what she was thinking *at the time* she was insulting me. What she was thinking was this: "This guy is great! I cannot believe he has not kicked me out of his office!" All the time she was insulting me, she was in fact admiring me. Again, this woman was exceeding bright. Why on earth would she act this way?

During the buildup to the third edition of the DSM, many psychiatrists came to the realization that these so-called "borderline" patients were not really "bordering" on psychosis at all. Patients who actually were on that border are now given other diagnostic labels in the DSM, such as *schizotypal*. Unfortunately, the name *borderline* still stuck for those patients I am now describing, creating the question (posed by Wynonna Ryder's character in the film *Girl Interrupted*), borderline between *what* and *what?* One researcher quipped that *borderline* is an adjective in search of a noun.

Before further discussing BPD, let me briefly define what a personality disorder is for those readers who do not know. To understand a full personality disorder, we must first define maladaptive personality *traits*. These are defined in the DSM IV as "enduring patterns of inner experience and behavior that deviate markedly from the expectations of the culture of the individual who exhibits it."

Maladaptive means that the trait must either create emotional distress for individuals or have some negative effect on their general everyday functioning. If, for instance, they drive other people to distraction, this quality might prevent them from holding a job for long. To qualify as a criterion for a personality *disorder*, the trait must also be persistent. That is, it should be present for most of the patient's adult life and have its origins in adolescence or even earlier. Furthermore, it must be pervasive, which means the trait should manifest itself in a significant number of different environmental or social contexts.

The trait does not, however, have to present in *every* environmental context. In fact, there are always contexts in which such traits do not manifest themselves. This is an extremely important point. If a repetitive behavior pattern is primarily a reaction to the individual's social environment and can be turned off and on at will, it is more likely to be primarily a psychological phenomenon rather that a physiological manifestation of a brain disorder. The fact that the maladaptive traits do not manifest in all social situations implies that people who have these traits may have some control over them and may have the ability to pick and choose when to engage in them and when not to.

In over thirty years of clinical experience with patients with BPD, I have seen BPD patients turn their aggravating behavior off and on like a faucet. The only time they cannot do so very easily is when they are in the course of a rage. Most people in a blind rage lose some control over themselves, so that fact does not really separate patients with BPD from the rest of us.

After I was able to figure out the tricks of the trade that allowed me to more easily deal with patients with BPD, I no longer witnessed the aggravating behavior much at all. In fact, most of the DSM BPD criteria appear and disappear in a given patient in an instant, depending on how the therapist acts and reacts. This fact alone makes the existence of some underlying biogenic brain disease state highly suspect.

We in the mental health profession share a tendency with most other people. Whenever we see people engaging in a pattern of behavior, we tend to attribute their behavior to their innate tendencies rather than seeing it as a reaction to the environmental situation with which they are dealing. Psychologists call the tendency to make this mistake the *primary attribution error.*[1] Several experiments in social psychology have shown that the environment is often the more important determinant; people's behavior is frequently shaped by and reactive to the social situations with which they are faced rather than solely by their innate tendencies.

Personality *disorders* are combinations of seemingly maladaptive personality traits that tend to occur alongside one other in many different patients at a frequency greater than one would predict by chance. For example, for BPD there are nine such traits. In addition to transient paranoid ideas, suicidal or self-injurious behavior, and anger control problems, BPD traits are frantic efforts to avoid abandonment, unstable and intense interpersonal relationships, unstable self-image, potentially harmful impulsivity, unstable emotions, and feelings of emptiness.

NOT A DISEASE

To qualify for the BPD diagnosis, a patient has to exhibit five or more of these nine criteria. This Chinese menu approach to personality disorders leads to some strange results. First, the cutoff number of five criteria is arbitrary. People who exhibit four of these criteria look a lot more like patients with BPD than do people with none of them. Second, one can have any five, six, seven, eight, or all nine traits. Doing the math, that makes 151 different combinations of traits that qualify a patient for the diagnosis.

Each trait may be mild, moderate, or severe, and one person who exhibits several traits of differing degrees of severity is not uncommon. In addition, once patients meet the criteria for BPD, they meet the criteria for, on average, between one and two *other* DSM personality disorders—*any* one to two of the ten other personality disorders. Clearly, despite their similarities, this is an extremely diverse group of patients.

Personality disorders are considered somewhat different from most other psychiatric disorders in that they have been, up until recently, assumed to be lifelong maladaptive psychological adaptations to the social environment rather than diseases. Almost all maladaptive personality traits that are listed in the DSM revolve around social behavior. For this reason, they are categorized on their own "Axis" in patient diagnoses, *Axis II.* (Axis III lists nonpsychiatric medical disorders, Axis IV environmental stressors, and Axis V is a rating of a patient's overall social and occupational functioning.) For some unfathomable reason, the diagnosis of mental retardation was also placed on Axis II, but I digress.

The personality disorders were divided into three *clusters*, named, rather uncreatively, *Cluster A, Cluster B,* and *Cluster C.* Cluster A disorders are the ones that actually border on psychosis; they are characterized by odd and eccentric behavior. Many of the patients who have the signs and symptoms of them may eventually fall victim to a schizophrenic breakdown. These disorders may therefore be prepsychotic conditions that are not really personality disorders at all. Borderline personality disorder is part of Cluster B, the erratic and dramatic personality disorders. Cluster C personality disorders are characterized by anxious, avoidant, or dependant behavior.

The behavior of patients with BPD is at times so extreme that psychiatrists who are biologically oriented have assumed that they must have some underlying brain dysfunction. In fact, differences in size and function of various part of the brain's limbic system in patients with BPD have been found. Once again, these differences are just assumed to be abnormalities when they could instead be conditioned responses or adaptations to difficult social environments.

Before discussing what might be going on in the brains of patients diagnosed with BPD, I will first look at three "deficits" in brain functioning that patients with BPD are thought by many to have. These deficits also conveniently appear and reappear at different times depending on what is going on in their relationships. Mental health professionals can easily appreciate this if they carefully listen to their patients and closely observe them.

OTHER NON-DSM CHARACTERISTICS OF BPD

One major characteristic seen in patients with BPD in mental health treatment centers is their apparent inability to see other people's good and bad characteristics at the same time. At times they react to others as if they are gods and then at other times as if they are nothing but piles of dung. If they at first seem to see the therapist as all good, they idealize the therapist and treat him or her like their personal hero. This behavior will continue for a while, but look out! An unsuspecting therapist will, without much warning, be knocked off his or her pedestal in a flash. The therapist will then suddenly be characterized by the patient as the aforementioned manure. This form of black-and-white thinking is called *splitting* by mental health professionals, and patients with BPD are assumed to lack the mental ability to integrate both good and bad attributes of others at the same time.

Psychoanalysts at first assumed, correctly I believe, that splitting was a defense mechanism. They believe that defense mechanisms originate because of experiences an individual has in early childhood with attachment figures, primarily the parents. Parents who mistreat their children cause a great deal of distress for them, and parents' cruelty is difficult for a small child to reconcile with his or her need and desire for a loving parent. Since very young children cannot handle the confusion caused by this problem, they tend to "split" off the good aspects of the parent when thinking about the bad aspects. This induces panic because they need a good parent, so theoretically they then quickly switch to thinking of the parent as all good. When the parent misbehaves, they may suddenly switch to the idealizing mode in spite of their being mistreated.

However, an opinion gradually took hold in psychoanalysis that splitting is not a defense mechanism but rather a mental *deficit*. This conceptualization holds that patients with BPD and similar personality structures really lack the ability to integrate good and bad images of other people, and of themselves as well, because they failed to negotiate a psychological developmental stage during toddlerhood. Based on the observations of a psychoanalyst named Margaret Mahler, this theory held that "normal" children learn to integrate good and bad images around the age of two, but fail to do so if their primary caretakers do not provide them with certain needs. How Mahler would know with that degree of specificity what was going on in the mind of a two-year-old is anyone's guess.

Nonetheless, many analysts still believe this. Of course, if they read the social psychology literature, and very few do, they would know that normal children have been studied in this regard. Three different studies[2-4] using three completely different methodologies all came to the same conclusion. Normal children first start to learn to integrate good and bad images of others at the average age of eleven and a half. They do not get particularly good at it until they are about fifteen.

I have seen my patients with BPD engage in splitting behavior many times, so the observations on which these ideas are based are not invalid. However, the times that they do *not* engage in it are, because of a theoretical blind spot, routinely discounted by clinicians. They engage in splitting and other provocative behavior primarily with parents, siblings, lovers, and of course doctors. With acquaintances and people they do not care much about, they do not really exhibit it much at all. I believe that the splitting behavior is part of their persona or false self.

I got into an argument with another psychiatrist about whether splitting was really just an act, stating my belief that while patients with BPD often act *as if* they lack this ability, clearly they have it. I told him that many times my patients, when they felt like it, could easily list the strengths and weaknesses of others at the same time. He retorted that this observation does not prove that they are able to integrate good and bad images of others. I had to ask myself, how on Earth could patients ever prove to him that he was wrong about them if the clear performance of a feat is not evidence of the capability of performing that feat?

Strangely, the same professionals who believe that BPD patients actually have this deficit often marvel at how successfully patients with the disorder can manipulate other people. If patients with BPD were not able to assess other people's strengths and weaknesses simultaneously, how could they successfully manipulate them? Anyone lacking this ability would fail miserably. In fact, patients with BPD are so good at reading other people and pushing their buttons that I never cease to be amazed by their extraordinary skills in doing so. When I first started to directly hear adult patients with the disorder interact with their parents, I was impressed by how easily my patients had been able to induce me to sound just like their parents.

Interestingly, mental health clinicians engage in splitting themselves all the time. When we think of, say, a child abuser, we tend to vilify him and seem to think that he acts horribly all the time. This is obviously not the case. Albert Ellis, one of the founders of a type of psychotherapy called cognitive therapy that looks at the irrational assumptions about the world that people routinely make, actually lists equating individuals' good and bad *acts* with their being good or bad *as people* as fundamental among those irrational assumptions.

A second thing to remember is that when people are furious with someone, or pretending to be, they seldom feel like talking or thinking about any of the good things that the object of their fury may have done. Likewise, when one is feeling really good about someone, or pretending to, one rarely thinks of his or her annoying qualities. We all do this. When therapists implicitly criticize patients with BPD for doing it, they are invalidating the patients' feelings. As we shall soon see, such invalidation is one of the primary triggers for borderline-like behavior.

This example of misreading the abilities of patients with BPD ties in with a second thing that is often said about individuals with the disorder. Marsha Linehan, one of the leading theorists regarding the origins and treatment of BPD, talks about their "apparent competence."[5] According to this view, people with the disorder may be able to appear quite competent in, say, being assertive in certain situations. In other situations where assertiveness would serve them well, they cannot seem to reproduce the behavior if their lives depended on it. Therefore the competence they sometimes exhibit must only be "apparent."

One again has to ask how one can demonstrate, through performance, a competency that one does not possess. I suppose someone could fake it for a short time, but sooner or later his or her deficits would become apparent. Also once again, how can someone who *is* competent but does not *act* competently in certain situations ever demonstrate an ability if any performance of the competency in question is discounted in this manner? Could it be that the *consequences* of being assertive in one situation are not the same as those in the other? Alternately or additionally, might patients with BPD have reasons to act as if they were incompetent?

On the issue of behavioral competencies, it must be said that faking incompetence is far easier than faking competence. This point was graphically illustrated in the true story behind the film *The Killing Fields* about the genocide in Cambodia during the late 1970s. During that holocaust, the Khmer Rouge murdered anyone with an education. Even wearing glasses could get one a death sentence. They were literally trying to return the country to Stone Age conditions. In the story dramatized in the movie, the protagonist is a doctor who survives by pretending to be an illiterate peasant. Acting incompetent in this way was, paradoxically, the most competent thing he could have done. He had clear motivation for pretending to be illiterate. If patients with BPD are faking incompetence, what would their motive be in that situation? I will answer that shortly.

The third now-you-see-it, now-you-don't characteristic of patients with BPD is their tendency to distort facts when describing their interactions with others. Many of their reported histories of being abused as children, which will be discussed shortly, are routinely discounted because patients with the disorder routinely seem to exaggerate or minimize details in their stories. They offer global judgments about people, leave out important details, use words in unusual ways, exhibit spotty amnesia, and provide confused or contradictory descriptions of events and people.

Once again, however, if therapists want to get the real story, they have to learn how to ask the right questions in the right way. If therapists are empathic, insist on blow-by-blow descriptions of various encounters rather than accepting global character judgments, and politely confront patients with inconsistencies and apparent holes in the stories they tell, patients with BPD can be induced to tell very accurate stories. Statements they make such as "he lies all the time" or "my mother is very controlling" can be very misleading and are therefore useless to the therapist for understanding the patient's social system. The therapist has to know what the alleged liar is lying about or exactly what behavior the patient thinks her mother is trying to control and how her mother goes about trying to control it.

The reader may ask: When I get a detailed story by doing this, how do I know the stories are accurate? I have found various means to get corroboration, or to observe interpersonal encounters directly. Before I describe these methods, I will first look at some evidence about the nature of the risk factors for development of the disorder.

RISK FACTORS FOR BPD

The borderline diagnosis is seen quite commonly today, with an estimated prevalence of close to 2 percent of the general population, and as high as about a fourth of all psychiatric outpatients. Despite this now being the case, these patients were considered relatively rare by psychoanalysts as recently as the mid 1970s, when I was in my residency program. Some psychiatrists think that perhaps, because they had not been extensively described in the literature back then, that mental health professionals were overlooking the syndrome. In other words, BPD behavior was being missed.

Overlooking these character traits? I am sorry, but with behavior such as that described earlier, they would be impossible to miss. Besides that, the traits would have been overlooked at a time when most psychiatrists were psychoanalysts who focused primarily on character traits. Patients with BPD were considered to be fairly rare, most likely, because they used to be—well, fairly rare. If true, that would mean that the incidence of new cases must have risen dramatically in the last thirty-five years.

Since the human gene pool does not change significantly in that period of time, and since we know of nothing in the water supply that would cause BPD, my guess is that something in our culture must have changed to cause this explosion of cases. Further evidence for this proposition is the fact that the diagnosis is rarely if ever seen in traditional cultures, such as those in rural India, but is starting to be seen in the more "modern" cities nearby. Truly biogenetic disorders like schizophrenia and bipolar disorder have about the same incidence in any population one looks at.

One of the support groups for the parents of patients diagnosed with BPD believes that this disorder is entirely caused by a biological abnormality and that dysfunctional families and child abuse have nothing to do with it. They have been lobbying the APA to move the disorder from Axis II to Axis I. However, a large number of studies are unanimous in showing that a history of child abuse is highly prevalent in reports about the backgrounds of individuals suffering with the disorder.

Of course, a significant percentage of individuals with the disorder were *not* physically or sexually abused, but as we have discussed, that is the case with any risk factor. Family dysfunction and child abuse are by far the most common of all biological, psychological, or social factors present in the background of patients with BPD seen in the literature today.

In an attempt to explain this away, some individuals have verbally offered the argument to me that BPD patients are different from birth. I have been told that if I had a child as aggravating as BPD patients are, I might be at risk for becoming abusive myself. I have heard similar arguments in regard to ADHD. One so-called expert presenting grand rounds at my school even attributed the increased incidence of alcoholism seen in the parents of ADHD children to the effects of having to deal with a difficult child. Difficult children are a cause of parental alcoholism? Children are responsible for their own abuse? Talk about blaming the victim!

In fairness, parental frustration with a difficult child probably does increase the odds that a parent who is already feeling overwhelmed, helpless, and besieged by unmanageable guilt might lose control and beat a kid. On the other hand, how do the people advocating this line of reasoning explain childhood sexual abuse? "She was so frustrating that I just had to rape her?"

FAMILY DYNAMICS OF BORDERLINE PERSONALITY DISORDER

When I first started practice, studies about the abuse histories in BPD had not yet been done, so nobody had any clue as to what created their odd behavior. I got my first whiff of the family dysfunction in patients with BPD quite by accident. In this instance I was also provided with a clue as to what might underlie borderline rage. Early in my private practice, I was referred the hospital case of a woman in her late teens. She was a strong girl, and when I first met her she was being dragged against her will into the ward by several burly psychiatric technicians. Before she had even arrived, I had heard that she had many episodes of rage and that she had broken almost every door and appliance in her house. As far as I knew, she had never hit a person.

I had had no training in family psychotherapy at all, but for some perverse reason I decided to have a meeting with her and her mother. During the meeting, an argument broke out between them. In a manner similar to my earlier experience with BPD rage, the girl suddenly started going into one. How did the mother respond? Instead of backing away prudently, her mother stuck her nose in the patient's face and started to berate her. Before I could do anything about it, the girl slugged her mother in the face as hard as she could. The aforementioned burly psych techs quickly returned and dragged her away once again.

I was far more fascinated with the mother's behavior than I was with the patient's. I knew the girl had violent tendencies, and I had only just met her. The mother had lived with her for years. Why would mom stick her nose in the patient's face and berate her when she was going into a rage? Ever hear of the expression, "She was asking for it?" As mentioned, the patient had never directed her rage against a person before. Later I learned that in the patient's home her sister would always find a way to distract the two of them before they ever got to that point.

Later I saw the mother herself as a therapy patient. I also briefly treated her sister and had a conjoint session with the patient and her father. I even saw the patient's boyfriend for a short time. Seeing the whole family separately and in various combinations created a sort of 360-degree view of the nature of their family interactions. I have since had many opportunities to have conjoint sessions with a patient and one parent, or to see a mother and her BPD daughter separately as therapy patients.

I even had the experience of supervising, using videotaped therapy sessions, one resident who was seeing the mother of an adult patient with BPD at the same time as another who was seeing the patient. Hearing the mother and daughter independently describe the same interaction from their own differing yet complementary perspectives led me to some fascinating insights about the nature of family-of-origin relationships in the families of patients with BPD. Still, I had no way to be certain that what I was seeing in the office was also happening in the family's natural environment.

By pure serendipity I had a chance to listen to such an interaction between a female with BPD and her mother. The patient was frustrated with the fact that previous therapists had not believed her stories and had accused her of distorting what she had been reporting about her relationships. To prove to me that she was telling the truth, she recorded a telephone conversation between her and her mother without letting the mother know that she was being recorded.

Since then, other patients have brought in such tapes, as well as letters written to them by their parents. Taping a conversation in this manner is illegal in some states, but my listening to them is not. Of course the patient knew that the conversation was being recorded, and she might have altered her behavior somewhat for my benefit, but if she had I would expect that the parent would notice that she was acting differently than she normally did and question her about it.

The first tape I heard showed indeed that the patient's description of her relationship with her mother was relatively accurate, but it also showed me that she had not told me the whole story. As I mentioned earlier, the first thing I noticed in listening to the tape was how often I had said things to the patient that were similar to what the mother was saying. I was very impressed that anyone could get me to do that with so little effort. A second thing I noticed was that the conversation went on and on for quite some time, with the same basic things being repeated over and over again ad nauseum.

The mother seemed to exhibit an almost compulsive need to offer the exact same advice repeatedly, and the patient seemed to compulsively give her opportunities to do so. Along with using many other fascinating techniques, the patient never clearly agreed or disagreed with anything the mother said. Despite being invalidated in this way, the mother persisted in giving her very much adult daughter the exact same advice numerous different times.

My first idea about the family dynamics of patients with BPD was that their parents might in general be extremely overinvolved with their offspring, and that this had something to do with why patients with BPD acted the way that they did. What appeared to be happening with the parents was similar to the changes in parenting practices that I described in Chapter Two, only multiplied by a factor of ten. They seemed to be trying to micromanage their children's lives.

Later studies did begin to show that some patients with the disorder indeed reported that their parents were overinvolved and overprotective when the patients were children and treated them as if they were incompetent. However, studies also showed that patients frequently reported some other seemingly dissimilar themes about their childhood family experiences, such as abuse, neglect, and a total abdication of the parental role by both parents that was termed *biparental failure.* I realized that the picture was a bit more complicated than I had first thought.

Other theorists besides me also began to notice odd patterns of behavior in the families of origin of patients with BPD, and a picture began to emerge. To make a long story shorter, what seems to be happening is that the parents of these patients *oscillate* between over-involvement and underinvolvement, and that in both instances much hostility is often, although not constantly, involved. The degree and pervasiveness of the hostility and the immensity of the swings between the two poles vary greatly from one family to the next and seem to have something to do with how severe a case of BPD their child exhibits.

In one extreme example of such oscillation, when one of my patients was a young teen, her father literally raped her one day and bought her a pony the next. Interpersonal psychologist Lorna Benjamin[6] speaks of sexually abusive fathers who, before the act, tell their daughters that they are the light of their lives. Afterwards, they tell the girls to go wash themselves because they are filthy whores. Of course, the parental behavior does not need to be anywhere near so extreme to be emblematic of the pattern I am describing. Also worth mentioning is that the parents do not necessarily act in this contradictory way with all of their children. Often only one sibling gets to be "it."

In a given family, either under- or overinvolvement may predominate, but if one waits long enough, the other polarity rears its ugly head. Child physical abuse and even incest result from the overinvolvement pole, while neglect and biparental failure result from the underinvolvement pole. Furthermore, even when parents are neglecting their offspring, they often blame their behavior on the child they are neglecting. What they say generally takes the form of something similar to "If you weren't such a horrible kid, I would not have to get away from you like this." From a child's perspective, they seem to continue to be completely focused on their children even while separated from them for extended periods.

In adults with BPD, these oscillations in attachment may lead to a sort of yo-yo effect. The BPD individuals move out, fail to make it on their own, and then get sucked back into the family. Soon thereafter the family gets irritated with them, performs "tough love" and throws the rascals out, only to later reel them back in once again to begin the cycle anew.

In some families the patients with BPD are ostensibly estranged from the parents, but infrequent but dramatic encounters between them nonetheless take place. For example, one patient in her forties told me at first that she no longer ever talked to her mother. Later she admitted that she had neglected to tell me about the monthly middle-of-the-night phone calls from the mother in which the mother berated my patient for being gay, but then concluded the conversations with professions of how much she loved her daughter. In still other families, otherwise uninvolved relatives relay messages back and forth between the patient and the parents.

These episodic interactions, I believe, reinforce a lot of the borderline symptoms because they induce a behavior that psychoanalysts refer to as *spoiling*. Because of the early learning tracts in the brain that are resistant to weakening and the variable intermittent reinforcement schedule process described in the last chapter, the problematic interactions do not have to occur very often at all to have tremendous power to trigger borderline behavior. The troublesome family behavior patterns can also be interspersed with other periods of much more pleasant interactions yet still create problems. The presence of the good times may in fact make matters worse rather than better, because individuals with BPD have even more trouble making sense of the parents' contradictory behavior than they would if the parents never acted in a loving manner. No wonder they sometimes engage in splitting.

Spoiling Behavior

After observing family dynamics of patients with BPD for years, I began to better understand an earlier observation made by the first psychiatrists to deal with patients who would later carry the BPD label. Followers of an analyst named Melanie Klein described the spoiling behavior pattern exhibited by them. Whenever a therapist tries to say or do anything helpful, the patient does something to spoil the effort and make sure that the effort fails. The effort is devalued, mislabeled, turned on its ear, or in some other way used to make the therapist feel useless, helpless, or angry.

Nothing the therapist does is appreciated by the patient, and instead the therapist might be accused of having evil or some other ulterior motives. Doing a favor for a patient with BPD outside of the office is often an invitation to be constantly harangued with more requests, or possibly even to be stalked, as was humorously but inaccurately portrayed in the movie *What about Bob?*

Klein thought that spoiling behavior had its roots in infancy and had something to do with primitive envy at the mother's breast. That interpretation made no sense to me and always seemed to me to border on psychotic. I just could never get my head around it. I believe that spoiling has more to do with a child's reactions to the oscillations in the behavior of the parents and the parents' complete preoccupation with and anger at their child. As I alluded to earlier, young children are not able to understand that parents can have mixed motives or confusion about what they expect from their children. Even after children learn how to seemingly meet the family's confusing demands, they nonetheless try to come up with their own explanation for them.

How do children understand their parents—and one theorist named John Bowlby said that children become experts on how their parents react at a very early age[7]—when the parents seem to make such contradictory demands? To answer that, I must first take a slight detour into a theory of the origins of BPD put forth by an analyst named James Masterson.[8] He believed that the parents of future BPD patients are somehow threatened when their children start to develop their own identity and no longer need their parents as much as they did when the children were babies.

Being a believer in Mahler, he believed that the main problem took place when a child was about two years old and first exhibited the early signs of developing autonomy. According to this view, when the child starts to gain some slight measure of independence at this age, the parents emotionally withdraw or abandon the child. To prevent the terror caused by the abandonment, the child then forms a compliant, inadequate false self to keep the parents connected.

I have to ask, however, if parents are threatened by the autonomy needs of a two-year-old, how must they react when the child reaches adolescence? Or when the child is old enough to move out of the parental home? I have seen clear evidence of emotional withdrawal by parents when my adult patients with BPD start to act more independently.

The autonomy issue ties into another feature of families of patients with BPD that Linehan describes. She theorizes that one of the two main causal factors that create the disorder, along with an inborn temperament that she presupposes causes future BPD children to have poorly regulated emotional responses, is what she calls an *invalidating environment*.[9] She does not actually refer specifically to the patient's family of origin as the invalidating environment, but what else this environment might consist of is hard to fathom. She defines invalidation as an erratic, inappropriate, and extreme response to an individual's communication of private experiences such as feelings, perceptions, or opinions.

In invalidation, such communication is attributed to the accused person's undesirable personality traits or socially unacceptable impulses. It is not simple disagreement with what a person says, but an indictment of the person's entire being. Individuals being invalidated are essentially being told that they are full of baloney, do not know what they are talking about or even how they really feel, or are perhaps completely insane.

I agree that frequent invalidating responses are characteristic of the families of patients with BPD. When powerful adults do this, children naturally start to doubt their own perceptions or even their own sanity. More important, I believe that the children eventually conclude that the invalidation is a reflection of the parents' *need* to believe that their child is incapable of making informed decisions about his or her own life and is unable do anything right. They notice that the parents routinely ignore evidence that such is not the case. The compulsive nature of the parents' invalidating behavior, when combined with the obvious parental blind spot, must mean, the child concludes, that the parents do not *want* the child to grow up. This further reinforces the child's earlier belief that the parents are totally preoccupied with him or her.

Invalidation involves another similar process known by communications theorists and linguists as *disqualification*.[10] People disqualify their own communication when they feel the need to communicate a feeling or opinion but are highly conflicted about doing so. They want to say something but are afraid to say it for fear that the person listening will attack them for it. Thus, they will not admit to having an opinion that they seemingly have just expressed. This legerdemain is accomplished by contradicting themselves in some very subtle ways in order to "take back" or divert attention from what had just been said.

The person may change the subject without seeming to have done so, change the meaning of his or her words from literal to figurative or vice versa, switch to a slightly different alternate meaning of his or her words, use obscure speech mannerisms, go off on tangents, or ask a question or statement with unspoken implications that contradict earlier meanings. All this is done without an admission that anything is amiss.

If, say, a young girl were to accuse her mother of hating her after a vicious attack by the mother, the mother might use these tricks to disqualify her own anger for reasons that will be explored shortly. The disqualification is actually something that the mother is doing to herself, because she does not want to admit, for example, how overburdened the child makes her feel, because this feeling does not fit with the mother's image of herself as a loving parent. The child unfortunately has no way of knowing about her mother's insecurity.

From the daughter's point of view, the mother's disqualification of her own communication looks like an invalidation of the daughter's observation regarding the extent of the mother's anger. Furthermore, it communicates to the child that the mother will not admit to any of her apparent needs to be preoccupied with her child, to not want the child to grow up, and to be angry at the child. One patient of mine reported an instance in which her mother had contradicted what she, the mother, had just said; when the patient pointed this out, she was immediately accused by her mother of "living in the past." In some families, questions about apparent double messages are met with more extreme responses such as physical violence. Children quickly learn that trying to discuss their relationship further is a waste of time and perhaps dangerous as well.

How does the child put all this together? To summarize, from the point of view of children trying to understand what the parents expect of them: On the one hand their parents seem to need them around and to be totally preoccupied with them, even when they neglect the children. On the other hand, their parents seem to hate them and resent any demands the child's presence places on them. How does a child then go about giving the parents what they need so that the child is not abandoned?

Spoiling behavior seems to be an ingenious and absolutely perfect solution. If a child becomes defiant, oppositional, a bit antisocial, incompetent, and acts in hateful and demanding ways with the parents, the parents get to have both of their seeming "needs" met. They can be preoccupied with the child, because the child is constantly getting into trouble and never seems to grow up and become independent from them. They also have been given an excuse to be angry and act in a hateful manner toward their child. Like some of the parents of patients with BPD occasionally say, "If you had a child like that, you might become abusive too." Having been the recipient of spoiling behavior from my patients with BPD, I do understand what they are talking about.

The examples I gave earlier of patients who were clearly trying to aggravate me are good examples of some of the tricks of the spoiler's trade. The false self of the patient with BPD is activated in any later relationship in which themes of dependency or personal adequacy might arise, or in cases of encounters with helpful figures who think they know more than the patient. The therapist-patient relationship is a prime example of just such a case. Patients can practice their spoiling skills with a therapist. Therapists ostensibly want to help the patient to act more maturely and be more competent, but how does a patient know if the therapist really might be scheming to make the patient dependent on therapy so the therapist can continue to bill for more sessions?

Perhaps that sounds like the patient is being hypersuspicious, but it ain't necessarily so. I have met therapists whose primary therapeutic goal was to keep patients in therapy as long as possible. This goal was rationalized with the idea that patients can never get too much therapy because they always have room for further personal growth.

At an academic psychotherapy meeting I once heard a presenter describe the case of a patient who had come for over two hundred sessions but had then suddenly dropped out. The presenter's conclusion about why the patient terminated her therapy? The patient was said to be "unable to form a relationship." In this particular professional group, one is supposed to show respect for different points of view, but I had to be restrained. I started to jump up and say, "She came to you over *two hundred times* and you think she *can't form a relationship*? Did it ever occur to you that maybe she felt that the therapy was not helping?"

The spoiler role, despite being played so compulsively, is anything but fun for patients. I believe that, because of the kin selection phenomenon, they continue to play it despite its being very ungratifying. Because they secretly hate the role, they covertly hope that therapists will not fall for their usual provocative maneuvers, although they will try fiercely to get them to do so.

Knowing about this ambivalence allows a therapist to respond in different ways that literally stop the patient in his or her tracks. The patient can be induced to stop spoiling with the therapist relatively quickly in all but the most severe cases. A problem remains, however, because these therapist interventions only work for that one relationship and do not carry over to any other of the patient's relationships. Therapists who deal with patients with BPD from all theoretical persuasions start therapy by using variations of these responses. A discussion of these interventions is beyond the scope of this volume but can be found elsewhere.[11]

Co-conspirators

Because playing the spoiler role is so difficult, patients with BPD will often enlist as intimates other people who can help them continue to play it. These helpful individuals, because of their own false selves, essentially feed into the spoilers' behavior as well as provide them with numerous opportunities to practice their false selves. What I am proposing here is similar to the twelve-step program concept of *enabling*. Enablers are cohorts of alcoholics called *co-dependents* who feed their habit, cover for them when they get in trouble, and engage in other acts that allow the alcoholic to continue to drink.

When two individuals feel the need to find partners who will help them maintain an ungratifying role, they will gravitate toward people covertly willing to serve this function. However, this is a two-way street. To stay with the enabler example, the co-dependent helps the alcoholic remain an alcoholic, but the alcoholic also helps the co-dependent to remain a co-dependent.

With patients with BPD, spouses are frequently individuals who attempt to help the spouse with BPD feel better while trying to tolerate the spoiling way in which the BPD spouse responds to their efforts. At the same time, they get angry at the BPD spouse for acting this way. Such individuals are frequently men who may qualify for the diagnosis of *narcissistic personality disorder*. Their behavior recreates for the person with BPD the family situation that produced the spoiling responses in the first place.

REGULATING A PARENT'S AFFECT: WHO IS TAKING CARE OF WHOM?

Getting back to the parents in cases of BPD, when adult children engage in spoiling behavior with parents, they are in a sense doing right back to the parents what the parents have done to them. They are invalidating the parents' attempts to take care of them. They give as good as they get. The spoiling behavior has become the child's false self, and more easily allows the parents to blame their anger on the child's behavior rather than attribute the child's anger to a valid feeling about the way he or she is being treated. However, if the child goes too far, the rage the parent begins to express may cause the parent to become unstable.

When the parents get too angry and start to become unstable, the children may then become alarmed. Although they believe that the parents need to be angry, they do not believe the parents want or need to be unstable. Furthermore, an unstable parent might be a danger to the whole family, and the family is what they are trying to protect in the first place. This reaction stems from the evolutionary forces of kin selection.

Spoiling behavior provides a solution to this quandary as well. Some types of spoiling behavior induce guilt in the parent, while others induce anger. When the parents become too angry, the budding borderline learns to make them feel guilty, and the parents' anger subsides. When the parents become too guilty and become unstable on that account—and guilt is part of what drives the parents' contradictory behavior in the first place, as we shall soon see—the borderline makes them feel angry, and the guilt subsides.

In my opinion, these children take it upon themselves to *regulate* their parents' emotional state. They will not usually admit this to anyone, because if a parent understood that to be what they were doing, they would not be able to do it as effectively. They have to make everyone think that their behavior is due to some defect or disorder that they have. To the outside world as well as to the family, the parents appear to be taking care of their incompetent children, while underneath the surface, the child is trying to take care of the parents' emotional needs. I refer to this shell game as "who is taking care of whom?"

In cases in which patients with BPD and their families spend most of their time at the overinvolved or *enmeshed* end of the overinvolved-underinvolved pendulum, this shell game can progress and lead to some very interesting behavior. A good example was the case of a man in his late thirties who still lived with his parents. He would rarely keep a job for long and was completely financially dependent on his folks. He often stole money from them and ran up significant bills on their credit card without permission.

Oddly, the parents always left money lying around the house in plain view, and never once called the credit card company to make sure that he would not be able to use the card again. They never once suggested that he move out. Whenever he offered to, they would tell him that he was too incompetent to make it on his own. Of course, they certainly had reason to believe that such was the case, but from the patient's point of view, they did this because they secretly wanted him to stay there and continue his seemingly outrageous behavior. The rest of the extended family criticized the patient unmercifully, and he never did anything other than give them more justification for doing so.

During his therapy, the other side of the "who is taking care of whom" shell game gradually emerged. The facts were these: the parents were elderly and lived in an extremely crime-ridden and dangerous neighborhood. Several other elderly residents had been burglarized and in some cases assaulted and almost killed. Almost all of the original inhabitants of the block on which they lived had moved out because of the escalating crime rate, but the patient's parents refused to budge. Furthermore, they were developing physical infirmities that made them easy targets and would act in careless ways that almost invited victimization.

The patient originally presented to me as a very angry and potentially explosive individual. Many of my office staff were fearful of him. In his neighborhood, he acted like a dangerous and possibly crazy fellow in many different and very public ways that communicated a strong message that he might go postal at a moment's notice. His behavior said, "Do not mess with me." In all probability, because of this behavior, his parents and their house were never touched by crime. Despite his angry appearance, he was in fact a highly fearful and nonviolent person. His false self had the desired effect of protecting his parents from crime while at the same time making it appear to the other family members that he was abusing them. He also seemed to most people to be completely dependent on them. His apparent "abuse" of his parents took place with their full cooperation.

This case illustrates another interesting point. With my patients, I have seen that if individuals with BPD think the parents need to invalidate them, they will do and say things that give the parents justification for doing so. They will act in juvenile, foolish, and hateful ways. In doing so, they in a sense invalidate themselves. They exaggerate, twist meanings, offer excuses, and in other ways disqualify their own communication so that no one will believe anything they say.

This may be the reason for the behavior of abuse victims discussed in Chapter Three, like the Roseanne Barrs of the world, who say things about their family that cannot possibly be true so that when they finally do tell the truth, no one gives them credence. They end up drawing anger and even hate onto themselves. Again, this is a difficult feat to accomplish and an even more difficult thing to experience on a daily basis. They nonetheless persist in the self-destructive and seemingly counterproductive behavior.

WHAT MIGHT BE GOING ON BIOLOGICALLY?

In Chapter Five, I explored the effects of social learning on the brain, and discussed how neural plasticity allows this to happen. In patients with BPD, several brain imaging studies have shown that certain parts of their limbic system are on average smaller, more active, or less active than those same parts in normal controls. The findings are somewhat inconsistent across studies, but likely they are real. For example, some but not all studies of the amygdala, particularly the left amygdala, show that it is on average smaller in size in patients with BPD than in control subjects.[12] As usual, most authors unthinkingly label this difference as an "abnormality," when it could in fact be a conditioned response that is highly adaptive in the BPD patient's social environment. We can understand what might be happening in the brains of patients with BPD by employing an idea called *error management theory*.[13]

In a chaotic, unpredictable, rapidly changing, and at times dangerous environment, reacting quickly to potential environmental dangers may help to prevent a disaster from occurring. If a person in such an environment overreacts when no danger actually exists, not much bad happens, but if a person does not react when danger is present, bad things follow. For example, if you run from what you think is a bear in the woods and it turns out to be a raccoon, the worst thing that happens is you get a bit out of breath for no good reason. On the other hand, if you do not run from what you think is a raccoon and it turns out to be a bear, you might just lose your life.

If the environment in which a person exists is chronically chaotic and potentially dangerous, the brain probably trains itself to do two things. First, it might very well train itself to be hypervigilant and to constantly be on guard against the worst possible scenarios. Second, it might train itself to err on the side of overreacting rather than erring on the side of underreacting. Becoming hypervigilant, expecting the worst, and having a tendency to overreact has survival value in this context, so the brain would reshape itself accordingly.

These are the very traits that patients with BPD exhibit in studies and in clinical situations. Social cues in particular, such as certain facial expressions, may be read somewhat differently by BPD subjects than by normal controls.[14] Some facial expressions are interpreted by subjects with BPD more negatively and less accurately than by normal controls. Other expressions are read in pretty much the same way as controls. With still other expressions, patients with BPD actually read them more accurately than normal controls.

Several such studies on the accuracy of reactions to different facial expressions in subjects with BPD have been done, and they seem to show contradictory results. The contradictions probably occurred because the environmental context in which the BPD subjects have grown up was not taken into account. In the type of family-of-origin environment I have described in this chapter, certain facial expressions signal far more potential danger to the family than others, so over- rather than underreacting to those particular expressions makes sense.

Patients with BPD tend to overreact, in my opinion, in order to prevent their bad family situation from getting worse. The family disaster they are trying to prevent might be family violence, increased drinking by alcoholic family members, or a threatened divorce by one of the family leaders. Being inhibited about responding quickly to the environment would lead to an increased likelihood of such deleterious effects coming to pass.

The brain contains both inhibitory neurons in circuits that slow down reactive behavior as well as excitatory neurons in circuits that speed it up. In individuals with BPD, the amygdala and other brain structures might be gradually shaped through ongoing environmental interaction so that inhibitory neurons that would be active under more normal circumstances decrease in number, leading to a decrease in the size of the structures and changes in the way they function.

We do not know if the changes that have been observed are reversible. If a psychotherapist is able to alter the family and psychological environment of the patient with BPD, and the changes are lasting, a good chance exists that they are.

WHAT MAKES THE PARENTS ACT THE WAY THEY DO?

The mystery of BPD cannot be solved solely by looking at the behavior of patients with members of their families of origin. That just moves the question of what causes BPD behavior from the individual to the parents. We need to understand why the parents act the way they do. In a type of psychotherapy known as Bowen family systems therapy, as well as in the type of therapy I use, the therapist investigates the relationships in the patient's family going back at least three generations, if possible, to see if the origins of and the reasons for maladaptive yet strongly ingrained family homeostatic patterns can be discerned. This emotional family tree is called a *genogram*.[15]

What I look for in the genogram are various experiences that have taken place as individual family members negotiated some of the major cultural changes that have taken place over the last several decades. Cultural trends as personally experienced by each important family member interact with other personal events, such as immigration from a foreign country that has different cultural values than does the United States, unpredictable death and diseases, experiences with racism and sexism, religious dogma, and many other factors. That leads families to adopt certain *family rules* that help the entire family adapt to their environment. These rules function to guide the behavior of each family member, and the behavior of members who break them is invalidated by the rest of the family. If the rule breakers persist, they may be disowned, subjected to violence, or in some cultures even killed.

Family rules are usually accompanied by *family myths*. Family myths function much like a religious dogma that predicts a terrible fate for anyone who dares break the church's rules of conduct. The family myths are often repeated frequently by family members in several different contexts through the use of slogans, proverbs, or common sayings in the culture such as "nice guys finish last," "the devil you know is better than the devil you don't," or "why would he buy the cow if he gets the milk for free?"

In many cases one family member volunteers to be or is recruited to be a rule breaker who, because he or she breaks the rules, meets with a bad fate—a black sheep who becomes a sacrificial lamb. For example, the "loose woman" in the 1930s who followed a disreputable career in show business might later indirectly kill herself by contacting syphilis or from drinking too much. Her fate proved the validity of the family myth about women who act on a desire for a career, and it helped to keep everyone else in line. Almost no one can remain a saint without the frightening example of a sinner to keep them honest.

As the cultural environment evolves, as we saw in Chapter Two, strong family rules often do not keep up with the times because of the phenomenon of cultural lag. Younger members of the family in particular, who usually interact in school with a wide variety of peers whose families have rules different from theirs, are often tempted to adopt behaviors that would, if acted on, create frightening negative family reactions. The Indian woman born in the U.S. mentioned in Chapter Five whose family had arranged a marriage after she had fallen in love with an American man and who committed suicide was a good example. Her being so distraught by the awful choice with which she was faced probably led to the suicide.

Personal experiences with such cultural events as the Rosie the Riveter phenomenon, also described in Chapter Two, may create a situation in which the parents themselves are highly ambivalent about family rules such as the limitations on women's career choices seen in some traditional families. Because everyone in the family seems to cling to the old rules so tightly, any family member who has such ambivalence will try to hide it, because each member of the family believes that all the other family members will not accept any new behavior.

This pattern can create the sad and ironic situation in which almost everyone in a family would secretly like the rules to change in a similar direction, but no one dares suggest it because everyone is unaware of how everyone else really feels. All of them think that they would be rejected if they did. Even if they do challenge the family rules, others in the family may think they are just trying to test everyone else, and react negatively in a way that invalidates the new behavior, even if covertly the others would be just as happy with the change. This behavior reinforces the view of the challenger that any challenge to the rules will be rejected by the rest of the family.

The family rules and personal experiences of a family member interact with one another. They also interact with the family members' own inherent or genetic personality tendencies, predilections, and desires. These predispositions can make the suppression of ambivalent feelings either easier or more difficult. A Rosie the Riveter who was inherently ambitious, energetic, and did not particularly like being around small children would have a much more difficult time sticking to outmoded traditional female gender rules than one who was not particularly ambitious and who loved to be around children. A woman who was not allowed to experience the work world during World War II might not feel very conflicted about remaining solely a wife and mother at all, because she had not been exposed as much to the alternative.

Because of all of the individual experiences and personality factors that operate on the family at a given place and time, widespread effects of major cultural changes on common family rules that lag behind them become highly magnified in certain families. In the example of the creation of massive parental guilt over problems created by two-career families described in Chapter Two, the intrapsychic conflict for some people can become completely unbearable and lead to drastic measures meant to contain it. The drastic measures can backfire and make the problem even worse than it might be otherwise.

In the families of children who grow up to develop BPD, the predominant intrapsychic conflict seems to be a severe conflict over the very role of having children. The parents indirectly act as if they believe that being a parent is the end-all and be-all of human existence, yet at the same time they feel overburdened and unable to indulge strong individualistic but covert desires because of the very presence of their children. This is why they are so preoccupied with their children yet at the same time so angry with them.

Gender role change is not the only focus of the mash of cultural trends, individual experiences, and personal predilections that create the massive conflict over raising children seen in the parents of patients with BPD, but it is one of the most common. This may be the reason the disorder was first seen, and is still at least in clinical settings more often seen, in females. The changes in women's roles, as previously discussed, were so massive and came about so fast that many formerly adaptive family rules became outmoded almost instantly. Interestingly, the proportion of males among individuals with the disorder coming to me for treatment has gradually increased over the years, perhaps suggesting that changes in gender role functioning are continuing to evolve.

Parents who harbor resentment toward the very presence of their children are often aware of this resentment, but it does not fit with their image of themselves. Experiencing the resentment adds to their already hypertrophied and unbearable sense of guilt, because they think that having such feelings means that they are bad people. Particularly if they have become abusive, but not just in those cases, some come to the belief that their children are *better off without them*. They cannot admit to others that they feel this way, because it might be perceived by others as an implicit admission of their covert desire to get rid of their kids.

A common way to solve this dilemma is for such parents to push their children away, especially after they grow up, through either subtle or not-so-subtle means. They do so without saying why they do what they do. This process is called *distancing*. Often such parents act in mean or difficult ways with their children, say hateful things, and make impossible demands on them in the hopes that the obnoxious behavior will make their children run for the hills. Of course they do so ambivalently because they really do want to be loved by their children and to be involved in their lives.

The complex and ingenious solutions that individuals devise for such impossible emotional conflicts never cease to amaze me. One common pattern is one I have seen in mothers of adult children who act helpless and constantly call up their offspring to help take care of some of their needs. The twist is that they consistently do so at times when it is most inconvenient for the kids to come, and they demand help with tasks that they could clearly either do by themselves or hire someone else to do.

When the children tell their mother that the time is inconvenient, she then lays ridiculous guilt trips on them or accuses them of not caring about her. Instead of this pushing them away as the mother hopes, the children often drop what they are doing and run over to the mother's house to comply with the request. In response, their attempts to do what is asked of them are then criticized by the mother as inadequate. This leads them to resent their mother, just as she feels she deserves, but they tend to continue to come and remain connected to her. They are simultaneously pulled in and kept at arm's distance, and yet they keep trying to please their mother. This sort of pattern is often what is actually being referred to when patients make statements like "Nothing I do is ever good enough for my mother."

The experience of one patient provides an extremely dramatic example of distancing. When he was a young teenager, his stepfather ordered his mother to have sexual intercourse with the boy so the stepfather could watch. She actually complied with this demand. Afterwards she immediately sent the patient off to foster care. The patient naturally believed that he was being blamed for what had happened and was being punished by being sent away. The therapist spent a fair amount of time convincing him that she sent him away for his own protection. She was apparently, for whatever reason, unable to stand up to her husband, and sending her son away was the only thing she could do to keep him out of harm's way. In this case, the patient actually was better off without her.

When Individuals with BPD Have Children

Their parents' emphasis on and ambivalence about having babies is not lost on adults with BPD. Some feel that their job is to have a lot of babies, while others act out the other side of their parents' ambivalence and not have any children at all. For the ones who feel they must follow the family rule that being a parent is one's major purpose on Earth, an even worse bind is created that can lead to even more severe borderline behavior in their children.

Since the false self of people with BPD is rife with apparent incompetence, their need to appear incompetent carries over to their parenting skills when they have children of their own. They become even more highly dysfunctional parents than their parents before them. They may literally give their children drugs or alcohol, leave them unattended, or hang out with unsavory characters who are bad influences on the children. If they think that their own parents need to believe that they are bad people through and through, they might become directly abusive to their children. At the same time, they are as preoccupied with their children as much as their parents were.

In some families, incompetence in playing the role of parent seems to serve another function: It allows the parents of the patient with BPD to hang on to the cherished parent role into their old age. In the last thirty years, a dramatic increase in the numbers of grandparents raising their grandchildren has taken place. Sometimes the parent in the middle also lives in the house, but often not. Between 1990 and 1997, the number of children living in grandparent-headed households increased by a whopping 66 percent.[16] This trend seems to be continuing to the present day.

The persons in the middle—the mother or father of the child— usually fall into one of three categories: they are antisocial and end up in jail (antisocial personality disorder is also a Cluster B personality disorder just as is BPD), addicts or alcoholics, or individuals with BPD who neglect or abuse their children. In fact, all of these three types of people exhibit significant Cluster B personality traits at one time or another, although in addicts the traits may seem to disappear if and when the addicts clean up.

Because the grandchildren appear to be in such danger, the grandparents feel that they simply must take over the rearing of the child, and of course there is a lot of truth to their viewpoint. From the point of view of their own children, however, they are just looking for an excuse to do so because, once again, they are obsessed with the parental role and cannot let go of it. I believe that the grandchild's parents are covertly abdicating their parental role *in order* to allow their parents to continue to be obsessed with children and complain about it. They are offering up their own children as gifts to their parents.

I was able to hear this type of thinking up close and personal in the case mentioned earlier in which one of my psychiatry residents was the therapist for the mother of an adult patient with BPD, who was raising her grandchild, while another resident was the therapist for the daughter. The sessions were videotaped. In one of the daughter's taped sessions, she discussed what happened when her child's custody was transferred to her mother. She said, in essence, that she believed that her mother really wanted to take over the care of the child, but she was still bothered by the fact that her mother complained about it so much. She also wavered back and forth between expressing a desire to raise her own child and stating that her child was better off without her and with being under her mother's care.

On the mother's taped session, she was discussing the same events from her perspective. She spoke of the joys of raising her grandchild and how it was making her relationship with her husband closer. At the same time she expressed anger at the daughter for leaving her with the child, and had difficulty trying to understand her daughter's contradictory behavior. She was certain that her daughter loved her child and appeared at times to be a capable parent, and just could not figure out why the daughter was so irresponsible at other times.

I saw a similar pattern during a TV newsmagazine story about grandparents raising grandchildren. Several of the grandmas who were interviewed waxed eloquently about how their grandchild was the center of their universe and how raising their grandchild was such a joy and how it gave their lives new meaning. At other times during the same interview, however, they complained bitterly about how, as elderly women, chasing after their grandkids made them *soooo* tired. Not that both of these statements cannot be true simultaneously, but I suspect that their grandchildren would find the two sentiments somewhat contradictory. If these women expressed them so readily to a TV news reporter, one can confidently wager that their grandchildren had heard them as well.

Family dysfunction is of course not limited to the type of family issues that I have been discussing in this chapter, and it can create a lot of other personality problems besides BPD. Other, far less dramatic but nonetheless highly significant problems can be created in children when parents have other devilish conflicts over their roles in life that they will not readily admit to for fear that they would be rejected by their own extended family. In my opinion, while treating the dysphoria and anxiety created by dysfunctional family interactions with medication has much value, in order to really help such patients in the long run, the underlying relationship issues must be addressed. This would of course be the focus of psychotherapy instead of "med management."

Unfortunately, many psychotherapists also concentrate almost entirely upon what is going on inside their patients' heads, instead of upon what is transpiring in their ongoing family relationships. In the next chapter, I will discuss the ideas expressed by different schools of thought within psychotherapy, and how they sometimes neglect the real and still powerful relationships in their patients' lives, while still trying to deal with the fallout created by those very relationships.

9

A Tower of Psychobabble? Today's Psychotherapy, the Idea of Mental Defectiveness, and Family Systems Issues

When medical students who were not psychology majors as undergraduates first learn about psychotherapy, many are highly skeptical. First, they are not even sure physicians should be doing it, especially for those patients who do not have a severe psychiatric disorder but instead have anxiety, dysphoria, or behavior problems that are caused primarily by problems in living. Psychotherapy does not seem like a "medical" procedure for people who are really "sick"; it looks more like something a school guidance counselor or a "life coach" should do.

Second, the theories about human behavior on which psychotherapy is based seem to them to be highly speculative at best, often containing seemingly dubious speculation and wild inferential leaps from observed behavior. Most important, at last count approximately 400 different recognized *schools* or models of psychotherapy treatment are being practiced, each one based on a somewhat different theory about human personality and behavior change, and some of which seem to completely contradict one another.[1] This number does not even include all the "biological" theories.

When I lecture about therapy to third-year medical students, who are by then working in clinical settings under an apprentice model, I try to address these concerns. First of all, I mention that physicians do not just treat diseases; they also treat pain and dysfunction. An athlete who strains a muscle in a football game does not really have a disease in the same way that a diabetic has a disease, yet doctors have no trouble treating the resultant pain so the athlete can quickly return to the field. Clearly, psychological pain and dysfunction can be at least as bad and in many cases far worse than physical pain or disability.

Second, psychosocial factors are addressed in many other fields of medicine. Good cardiologists, for example, must help their patient quit smoking, change their diet, and get more exercise. In psychiatry, however, psychosocial factors take on much greater significance than they do in other fields because our organ of interest is the brain. As I have pointed out, the thinking parts of the brain responsible for psychological states and adaptations to the environment are highly intertwined with other parts of the brain. Although treating someone who is depressed with medication is extremely important, part of the doctor's responsibilities includes getting the patient off the medications eventually if possible and teaching the patient to cope with environmental stressors that may trigger future episodes if not addressed.

As for the many competing theories of human psychological functioning, several factors led to this situation. First, psychology is a relatively young science, and in any young science competing theories espoused by dogmatic theorists are the rule rather than the exception. In the not too distant past, physicists offered widely differing theories of what electricity was. As we learned more about the phenomenon, one theory eventually gained supremacy.

Second, the subject matter of psychology—human consciousness, perceptions, emotions, and cognitions—is not subject to direct observation. We cannot read minds, and as I have argued, when you ask people why they do what they do, they may not know, they may lie to you, or they may lie to themselves. We also cannot compare psychotherapy treatments using a double-blind procedure and with proper scientific controls, for all the reasons discussed in Chapter Six.

Last but hardly least is that human behavior is just so damned strange. When we look at self-injurers or hear stories about patients like those described in the last chapter, we shake our heads. Another anecdote I share with the students concerns a newspaper story I saw some time ago about a woman who repetitively extorted money from her own parents by faking her own kidnapping and demanding a ransom.

What was fascinating about the story was that the parents continued to pay off the ransom demands even after the police told them what she was up to. They eventually went broke and the father died of a heart attack, which is what led to the story making the papers. What did the woman do with all the money? She used it to buy drugs not only for herself but also for all of her many friends. I tell the students that if they think that heroin can make someone act that way, I have some oceanfront property in Arizona that I would like to sell to them. No wonder there are 400 different explanations for human behavior!

Despite the fact that so many different schools of psychotherapy exist, the problem is not quite as big as I am making it out to be. The 400 or so different schools fall into five major categories and two or three minor categories, each with its own primary themes and focus. These larger categories of schools splinter into subcategories on the basis of theoretical splits about the meaning, importance, and origins of some common behavioral patterns that are usually observed in the context of psychotherapy. Some of the resultant arguments really split hairs, devolving into debates much like the old theological argument about how many angels can dance on the head of a pin.

Each "theory" is not a single theory at all but a large collection of different ideas that share common elements. Despite the common elements, some of the ideas in each school of thought may be completely on target, while at the same time other parts are completely wrong. We now know, for instance, that the old psychoanalytic belief that harsh toilet training causes obsessive-compulsive disorder later in life, although still espoused in some corners, is empirically incorrect. This does not mean, however, that the whole psychoanalytic concept of defense mechanisms is also invalid.

Likewise, each school of psychotherapy employs many different interventions. Some of these interventions may be crucial, while others may be unnecessary or even counterproductive. Studies that show which parts of a treatment are necessary and which are superfluous are few and far between. Furthermore, even if interventions are shown to be effective, this does not prove that the theory that led to them is true.

I believe that almost all of the schools of thought in psychotherapy have something valid to say about the workings of the human mind, interpersonal relationships, and the processes by which they can be changed, while none of them offers a complete picture. If one listens to the leaders of each school and to many of those who teach the theories in psychology training programs, they seem to all be speaking different languages, like the people in the mythical tower of Babel. These leaders in the field seem to think that their theories explain everything about human psychology and that competing schools of thought are complete rubbish.

In actuality, the schools of thought all overlap considerably. In some instances, they are just calling the same exact phenomena by different names. In most instances, their argument is only about precisely what the phenomena mean. Many of these debates can be resolved by looking at all available sources of data: clinical anecdotes, RCTs, experimental psychology, cultural trends, and data from other disciplines such as social psychology, sociology, anthropology, neurobiology, genetics, and linguistics. Observations about what transpires in the mass culture and throughout human history are also important.

A complete description of all the major schools of psychotherapy is beyond the scope of this volume. I have listed two books in the references with more complete descriptions.[2] Here, I will greatly simplify the five major therapy school categories in order to briefly summarize how they conceptualize psychological problems that I believe are triggered primarily by dysfunctional family-of-origin interactions. I will also discuss how the proponents of many of the schools seem to believe that people who have psychological problems have some sort of mental defect or deficit. No doubt purveyors of the various schools will accuse me of oversimplifying their ideas and omitting subtle distinctions. However, I believe that the subtle distinctions are often what get in the way of efforts to integrate the various ideas. In the next chapter, I discuss integrating the schools with one another and with biological psychiatry, a process I again believe must involve extensive consideration of dysfunctional family relationships.

I will not be discussing any psychological theories about the origins of mental illnesses that are, in my opinion, clearly due primarily to pathological brain diseases, such as schizophrenia. Psychological theories about episodes of major mood disorders, as manifested when the patient is not in the euthymic state, are also excluded. I believe that primarily psychological explanations for these disorders are mostly nonsense, although social tension can make them worse, as can any form of stress. Medications remain the best available treatment for these disorders, despite their side effects and other risks.

PSYCHODYNAMIC PSYCHOTHERAPY

I have already discussed some of the ideas from the first and oldest category of therapy schools, psychodynamic psychotherapy, in earlier chapters. These therapy schools branched off from Freudian psychoanalysis. I discussed how the model of intrapsychic conflict is at its core, but how it has changed somewhat from a conflict model to more of a deficit model.

A central precept of psychoanalysis is that the conflicts that cause the most important psychological and behavioral problems arise in early childhood during different phases of psychological development. Analysts once took the position that personality is completely formed by the time an individual is five years of age. For example, during the so-called oral stage of early infancy, the infant's primary job in life is to learn how to feed and bond with his or her caretaker. If the baby cries because it is hungry and turns toward the mother's breast, a good-enough mother will be attuned to the baby's needs and provide the baby with a breast or a bottle. If instead she hits the baby over the head with a two-by-four, the baby just might develop conflicts and inner turmoil over its needs to feed and to bond. Hey, it could happen. I am only slightly exaggerating for effect.

Analytic theory then goes on to suppose that the baby is overwhelmed by the anxiety created by its need to feed and to bond and that in response the conflict becomes unconscious, so that later in life the child has an approach-avoidance conflict of which he or she is unaware over such things as bonding with potential intimates. Adults thusly affected will theoretically do one of two things. First, they may repeatedly become attached to abusive confederates. Second, they may make a compromise by maintaining distant relationships with a "safe" attachment figure. By safe I mean that the relationship will be characterized by a lack of true intimacy and commitment. A common example is women who have prolonged affairs with married men who always promise to eventually leave their wives but almost never do.

Again, some of the specific ideas about different stages and what transpires may be wrong, but the idea that intrapsychic conflict based on one's experiences in one's family of origin leads to maladaptive behavior has much merit. The idea that human beings use defense mechanisms in attempts to ward off unwanted aspects of themselves is clearly observable. That people often repeat the same dysfunctional behavior over and over again, often recreate the childhood environment from which they came, and often act toward others as adults in ways analogous to the way they interrelated with primary attachment figures such as parents (transference) are all readily observable phenomena.

I do have several issues with the therapeutic emphasis in psychoanalysis, and here I will focus on four of them. First, while early childhood experiences in one's family of origin are clearly important—remember those impossible-to-extinguish early fear tracts in the amygdala—we now know that the brain continually changes throughout life. We can learn to override those early fears and react using our intellect instead of our gut. If later interpersonal experiences could not alter dysfunctional character traits because the traits are already written in stone, then psychotherapists would be wasting their time. They would never be able to change a patient's habitual way of responding to the social environment.

In fact, psychoanalysis supposedly works through an analysis of transference, which is the way that character traits play out in the patient's relationship with the analyst in the here and now. Somehow, analysts have the chutzpah to think that their relationship with the patient has more power to affect the patient's behavior than the ongoing relationships that the patient has with his or her primary attachment figures. As I have argued, the latter relationships have a lot more power than any other relationships. This does not mean, however, that other relationships have no power at all.

The second issue I have with the analysts is one I have with many of the other schools. They tend to assume that their patients are incredibly stupid. In a sense, one could say that these theories presume that maladaptive behavior is caused by some sort of mental defect or deficit that blocks people from employing their normal intelligence to solve interpersonal and psychological problems. Thus most schools of psychotherapy, in order to explain problematic behavior, replace the biological defects presumed by biological psychiatrists with psychological defects.

To go with the example of the person who serially picks abusive partners, analysts tend to think that these patients are unaware of their own anxiety about intimacy and furthermore that they truly believe that all potential intimates will be abusive. In fact, such individuals are well aware of counterexamples of nonabusive relationships and purposefully ignore them.

People who continue to do the same problematic thing over and over are said by analysts to have a *repetition compulsion* that causes them to continually recreate the ungratifying consequences of their early childhood environment. One analytic theory is that they do this in the vain hope that they will gain "mastery" over the initial problematic family interactions. The problem with this explanation is that they would learn, after several failures to achieve mastery, that their efforts were doomed to failure. Albert Einstein is quoted as having said something like "The definition of insanity is doing the same thing over and over and expecting different results." Are people really too blinded by their own anxiety to notice this? I would think that the adverse consequences and the resultant pain this behavior brings on them would make the negative consequences rather conspicuous.

Many people clearly do repeat the same maladaptive behavior over and over again. In fact, the question of why they do so could be considered one of the two most important questions about human psychology that all psychotherapy schools try to answer. Because it is such a tricky question, attributing the repetition compulsion to people being inherently mad, bad, or stupid is easy. In other words, these people must be mentally defective. (The second question that the different therapy schools try to answer is that of how to get people to stop repeating problematic behavior and change it to something more gratifying.)

I believe that understanding the repetition compulsion lies in the answers to a question first posed by psychoanalytic pioneer Alfred Adler: What adverse consequences would ensue if such individuals *stopped* repeating the behavior? A desire to try to avoid any consequences that they perhaps envision cannot be motivated by selfishness, because pain is not pleasure. I have argued in this book and elsewhere that the adverse consequences they are attempting to avoid are certain negative effects on the rest of their family.

Another bone that I have to pick with psychoanalysts is their emphasis on individuals' *fantasies* about their relationships rather than on the real relationships. In analysis, other people are referred to as *internalized objects,* or *objects* for short. This does not mean that analysts think of other persons as things. The "object" here refers to the objects of the person's libido or, in other words, the objects of his or her affection and antipathy. *Object relations* refers to how the internal view of others and the internal view of oneself interact, as if what the other person is doing in reality does not really matter.

This emphasis shares its roots with a philosophy called *constructivism.* The most radical form of this philosophy proposes, in essence, that the only reality that exists is that which occurs in our minds. How we construe the outside universe is reality. Of course, in a sense this is true, because all of our ideas about the outside world exist inside our head, and we can never truly get inside another person's brain and experience what he or she experiences. The question is: How accurate are our constructions?

Analysts tend to think they are all distorted, as we discussed in the chapter on BPD. I, on the other hand, have found that when I ask nonpsychotic patients to role-play the behavior of their significant others, they are very good at predicting how the other will behave under a variety of circumstances. The longer they have known someone, the better the predictions are. The only things patients cannot predict is how the others will respond in situations that are completely novel in the patients' experiences with the other person. The ability of intimates to predict one another's behavior under a variety of external contexts far surpasses the ability of any psychological test to do the same. After all, if someone has been married for a number of years, he or she does not wake up to a different stranger every morning.

One last area of disagreement I have with psychodynamic therapy is that some therapists seem to think of their patients' spouses as a sort of enemy of the therapy. Spouses are often felt to be "subverting" the patient's psychotherapy when in fact they interfere because they have a valid interest in how the therapy turns out. They are viewed by analysts as wanting to keep the patient from changing only because of their own neurosis. A better understanding of a spouse's behavior in this regard will be described in the section on family systems therapy.

BEHAVIOR THERAPY

The second major category of psychotherapy schools is called *behavior therapy.* The initial purveyors of the theories behind this type of treatment dismissed any attempt to understand what happens inside the human mind as unscientific, precisely because we cannot read minds and therefore subjective mental experiences cannot be measured. Science, they believed, should concern itself only with things that can be measured. Everything else should be considered a *black box,* which is sort of like a black hole in that you cannot see inside of it directly and therefore cannot know what is going on in there. You can only see and measure inputs and outputs. This stance essentially eliminates all of subjective experience from scientific scrutiny, which to me is a very strange step to take indeed.

Behaviorists are called that because the psychology experiments from which they derive their theories and therapies are based on the observation of the behavior of animals, and in some cases the behavior of human beings. These scientists measure and quantify what animals actually do, as well as the environmental circumstances under which they do it. Unlike biological psychiatrists, they correctly ascertained that most mammalian behavior is not instinctual but learned, so they developed *learning theory.*

They first observed that animals exhibit a lot of different spontaneous behavior. Some of it seems to be "saved" and repeated while other behavior disappears never to be seen again. Environmental events that lead to either an increase or a decrease in the frequency that these behaviors are emitted are called *reinforcers,* and the process through which they operate to create learning is called *conditioning.*

The frequency, nature, and timing of the behavior-changing environmental events, as well as unmeasurable internal states of the animal at the time of the events such as how hungry it is (oops, what happened to the black box?), determine the power of the environmental reinforcers as well as whether they lead to an increase or decrease in the frequency of the behavior being studied. To boil things down, behaviorists see learning as created by environmental rewards and punishments for behavior. According to this view, maladaptive repetitive behavior is just the result of having learned bad habits. It is as simple as that. If a therapist wants a person to change, he or she has to find a way to remove the rewards or punishments that continue to reinforce the bad habits and then teach the patient good habits, which must then be shaped and reinforced through new rewards and punishments.

Learning theorists used animal models such as the behavior of rats in mazes and dogs in cages. They then in many cases extrapolated these results to human behavior. The reader may ask, is it accurate to extrapolate results in animal models to humans? Human beings have some talents that all other animals lack: enhanced learning ability, long memories, speech, thinking, and the ability to anticipate future consequences of behavior and change it accordingly. As they say, monkeys will never be able to compose a symphony.

Radical behaviorists such as the late B. F. Skinner, although thankfully diminishing in influence rapidly as we speak, answer the extrapolation question in the affirmative. They seem to believe that human thought is astonishingly unimportant, that human behavior is totally at the mercy of environmental reinforcers, and that humans somehow are not able to proactively change their own environment unless having been previously reinforced for doing so.

Once again, they are in a sense saying that people are defective in that they always react to their environment unthinkingly. This is patent nonsense. If true, it would mean paradoxically that Skinner believed his theories to be true only because he had been rewarded for thinking so, perhaps by his own professors. His theories would not have been based on conclusions formed through thoughtful consideration of the experimental evidence, and therefore their validity would be highly suspect.

Clearly, external rewards and punishments do affect our behavior, and this fact is often overlooked by psychoanalysts who focus mostly on internal processes. The biggest problem that I have with many behaviorist formulations is that they put more stock in nonhuman environmental reinforcers like food pellets or electric shocks than they do in the reinforcing power of the behavior of our fellow human beings. Humans are among the most social of all organisms, so one might think that events such as hearing your mother lay a guilt trip or being validated or invalidated by your family for your life choices would be more powerful environmental reinforcers for shaping human behavior than food or even sex.

When asked about self-destructive behavior, which would seem to run counter to their theories, extreme behaviorists immediately cop out by invoking the black box. They say they do not know why some of the behavior of certain individuals increases in frequency when they feel pain, when by all rights pain should function as a punishment rather than a reward and decrease its frequency. Still, human children are notorious for telling their parents, "I don't care what you take away from me or how much you spank me, I will not do what you tell me." This does not happen so much with rats receiving electric shocks.

In fairness, we do know that SIB can lead to the release of chemicals in the brain called endorphins, which are similar to drugs like morphine and which calm an individual down. Therefore what should be punishing—pain—may be overridden by the positive effect of the anxiety relief. This seems like a strange neurophysiologic mechanism to have been selected for through evolution. If one looks at individual organisms, it would seem to lack adaptive value. Perhaps, once again, we have to look at kin selection. Some SIB does occur in "normal" individuals under some cultural circumstances. For instance, in the festival of Ashura, Shia Moslems march down the street cutting their foreheads with razor blades or flogging themselves until they bleed.

Still, the consequences of self-destructive behavior should not function as a reward. Pain is not pleasure. This seeming paradox can be resolved if repetitive and painful self-destructive behavior leads to a decrease in even more painful anxiety because it seems to help the families of those that engage in it. This may be the mechanism through which the genetic force of kin selection exerts its influence on specific human behavior at the individual level.

The focus of behaviorists on animal models and nonhuman environmental events leads them to the conclusion that, in order to function as strong reinforcement, a reward or punishment needs to occur very close in time to the behavior that it affects. In humans, this is only partly true. Because of our long memories and those old familiar fear tracts in the amygdala, events that transpire in one's primary attachment relationships can continue to exert effects for a long time afterwards, often for years.

Continually giving in to the perceived demands of the family of origin can relieve anxiety, and it is that relief that may function as reinforcement. This type of reinforcement pattern is called *negative reinforcement*, and it is often confused with punishment. Negative reinforcement is what happens when an ongoing aversive stimulus is *terminated*, and it leads to an increase in the behavior that led to the termination. Punishment is the provision of an aversive stimulus rather than its termination, and it leads to a decrease in the behavior that led to it. Negative reinforcement is more powerful than reward in human behavior, and punishment for us is the least powerful reinforcer.

COGNITIVE THERAPY

Many academic psychologists were not happy about the behaviorists excluding mental life from studies in psychology. They asked themselves this: In some people, an experience such as being bitten by a dog just once leads to the development of a dog phobia. In others, multiple bites do not lead to such a development. What distinguishes the first person from the second? The two people are both exposed to a stimulus, a dog bite, which we will call A. Their response, either phobia or no phobia, cannot be B. The response must be C. An intermediating variable must exist to account for the difference between the first person's response and the second person's. What might that variable—the B in the formulation—be?

The psychologists postulated that the intermediating variable is cognition: thought or belief. What determines whether or not a human develops a dog phobia after being bitten is not just the experience of having been bitten but how the individual evaluates the dangers involved when again confronted with a dog. If the person thinks, "Omigod, I'm sure to get bitten again! The pain will be unbearable! I can't afford the medical treatment! I'll lose time from work and my boss will fire me! I'll end up broke and penniless in the gutter!" then surely he or she will be very frightened in the presence of any dog. I again exaggerate only slightly for effect. On the other hand, if the person thinks, "Last time I was bitten, it was by a Doberman pinscher that was barking at me; this is a toy poodle that is wagging its tail. Besides, I was trying to rob the owner's house when I got bitten before," then surely he or she will not be frightened.

Aaron Beck, one of the founders of cognitive therapy, initially studied depressed people and examined the depressing thoughts that they were thinking. He noticed some very interesting things.

Depressed people make a lot of logical errors when they think about both their current situation and their future. Furthermore, the exact same types of logical errors are made by many other depressed people. These thoughts come to the depressed person unbidden and automatically, so they came to be known as *automatic thoughts.* Furthermore, the thoughts are sort of subconscious—though heaven forbid cognitive therapists should use that word and sound too much like psychoanalysts—under the radar, so to speak.

Depressed individuals make logical errors such as *overgeneralizing.* This means that they think that just because something bad has happened once that it is bound to keep happening again and again. They *catastrophize,* which means they scare the heck out of themselves by imagining worst-case scenarios. They also set impossible goals for themselves and then flagellate themselves when they cannot meet them: "I must be valedictorian of my class or I'm no good at all!" This latter type of thinking came to be known humorously as musterbating or shoulding all over oneself. Many other types of logical errors rampage through their minds.

These therapists reasoned that if people could be taught to examine their own thinking critically and learn the logical errors of their ways, then they would approach their world more reasonably and not have unpleasant reactions such as chronic depression, anger, or anxiety. Cognitive therapy was the result. The therapist and the patient engage in a process known as *collaborative empiricism.* They look at the evidence. Just how likely are those worst-case scenarios they imagine? What god mandated that they must be valedictorian? If they flunked a test, maybe it was because they had not studied, and they were not doomed to continue flunking tests forever as they predict.

Cognitive therapists found that automatic irrational thoughts are not limited to depressed people, but that everyone engages in them at one time or another. This irrational thinking frequently leads to strong but unnecessary emotional responses that drive maladaptive behavior and chronic unpleasant feelings. I have no doubt that such is indeed the case. After all, if looking for irrational thinking in human beings is your task, you have a rather easy job. For example, why are some people afraid to fly in an airplane but refuse to put their baby in a car seat while driving? Which of those two contingencies is more likely to lead to a bad outcome? Having patients examine their own thinking can and frequently does have very beneficial effects on their mental outlook.

The question that arises is *why* people engage in illogical thinking. When asked, the cognitive therapists answer that we are just born that way. We are all just naturally stupid, I guess. Again, they are proposing yet another type of mental deficiency. Of course, some fears are hard-wired into our brains and are therefore instinctual, like fear of snakes, so on that level we may be at times naturally irrational. But are we really that stupid all the time?

A clue to the answer to this question can be found by looking at people who have personality disorders. Some of them, when confronted by the illogical nature of their thoughts, dig in their heels and say, "My mind is made up; don't confuse me with the facts." For example, one patient with BPD engaged in the usual "splitting" persona, trying to convince me that she was worthless because she could do absolutely nothing well. In response, I tried a psychotherapeutic technique known as *reframing*. Every time she came up with a new weakness that was supposed to characterize her, I would point out how the trait was actually strength in many contexts. I would redefine her stubbornness, for instance, as persistence.

The problem with my tactic was that she was much better at making lemons out of lemonade than I was at making lemonade out of lemons. Each and every time I tried to reframe some attribute of hers as a positive one, she was able to redefine it as negative. Finally, I said in frustration, "You're really good at that. I'm impressed. No matter what I point out about you, you can figure out a way to turn it into something bad." Her reply? "Oh, sure, the *one thing* I'm good at . . ."

Another common thought expressed by less disturbed patients is a bit more honest. They say, "I *know* what I am thinking is not rational, but I just cannot stop thinking it." I saw a videotape of Aaron Beck at work. His patient was saying precisely this. Beck acted as if he did not hear what the patient had just said. He went right on disputing the logic of the patient's thoughts and continued to ignore the fact that the patient was repeating, "I know that already." The other big name in the field, Albert Ellis, said that such people are taking their new rational beliefs "lightly," whatever that means.

When people hang on to a belief no matter what the evidence is against it, I believe that they are doing so deliberately at some level, no matter how much they protest that they really do believe what they are saying. Ignoring obvious information that conflicts with a belief takes mental effort. Another psychoanalytic pioneer, Karen Horney, postulated that these cherished ideas are what she called *security beliefs*, which she believed to be hallmarks of a false self. Security beliefs are formed to help an individual fit in with a family that seems to demand certain types of responses while punishing others. I have found that these security beliefs are identical in content to the family myths that I wrote about in Chapter Eight.

I believe that repetitive automatic irrational cognitions are meant to force the true self of an individual into toeing the family's party line. People who engage in this type of thinking are literally attempting to kill off or *mortify* a natural part of themselves that does not fit with perceived family needs. The irrational thoughts function as defense mechanisms. Albert Ellis would spin in his grave if heard me say that, but the evidence is there. I have had several experiences similar to the one I had with my previously described first patient with BPD who admitted far into therapy that she did not really believe the negative things about me that she had been insisting she believed for months. Some of my patients have admitted knowing things they had long insisted they did not only after years of therapy.

Automatic thoughts are automatic because people have trained themselves to react the way they do to the point where the thoughts that help them do so become habitual and come to them without conscious deliberation. In this sense, they are "unconscious." If we had to think about everything we do, we would be paralyzed. However, at some level, we are aware of what we are doing. Again, lying to oneself takes mental energy and cannot be a passive process, no matter how good an actor someone may be.

For many years cognitive therapists argued with experiential therapists, the therapy school discussed in the next section, about whether every human emotion was preceded by a cognitive evaluation of the environment. Cognitive therapists argued that such was always the case. Fortunately, brain science has evolved to the point where we can now answer that question. While complex emotions are indeed preceded by an evaluative thought, so-called "gut" emotions are triggered in our social early warning system in the amygdala, anterior cingulate, and other limbic brain structures. These brain circuits fire before the thinking parts of the brain have a chance to chime in. Such circuits can in a very short time later be overridden by the thinking parts of the brain. This is a good thing. If it were not true, providing psychotherapy would be a fool's errand. Some of what psychotherapy does is to try to slow automatic gut responses so patients have time to think about how they would like to react in certain situations.

Cognitive therapy and behavior therapy are relatively easy to combine. The therapist can look at bad habits, environmental reinforcement, and automatic thoughts to come up with a more broadly based formulation of a patient's problems than can be had by looking at any one of these factors alone. The combined form is called cognitive-behavioral therapy or CBT. I mentioned it earlier in the section on psychotherapy research. My biggest beef with CBT is that, in its traditional form, it neglects the power of interpersonal processes and family loyalty.

In actual practice, however, when CBT therapists treat people with significant personality disorders, a lot of what they do looks more and more like relationship-oriented psychodynamic therapy than it does like traditional CBT. They even deal with transference, although none of them dares call it that. In a training videotape shown in my residency program, one of the originators of CBT named Donald Meichenbaum was clearly seen drawing a parallel between a female patient's current relationship with her husband and her earlier relationship with her father. Marsha Linehan, the psychologist who coined the term *invalidating environment*, is also in the CBT camp.

EXPERIENTIAL/HUMANISTIC PSYCHOTHERAPY

The fourth major category of psychotherapy is called humanistic or experiential therapy, founded by Carl Rogers (*client-centered therapy*) and Fritz Perls (*Gestalt therapy*). This class of therapy has fallen somewhat out of favor for psychologists, possibly because of the excesses of the encounter group movement, which arose from Gestalt therapy at a retreat called Esalon in Big Sur, California, in the late 1960s and 1970s. Nonetheless, its techniques have survived because they are very powerful and are used not only by psychotherapists but also by industry trainers to change the behavior of members of a company's work force. If you have been a victim of a company's "trust-building exercise," for example, then you have been exposed to an *experiential* behavior change technique.

Both Perls and Rogers accepted Freud's intrapsychic conflict model but objected to the way the analysts divided up people's minds into parts like the id and superego. If a person was conflicted, they believed that the whole person was ambivalent. No warring parts of a self needed to be invoked. The humanistic therapists thought of people as whole (*holistically*). A mentally healthy person was thought to be one who felt free to express his or her true inner self and not have to kowtow to other people's ideas of what he or she should be or do, although one could take other people's desires into account. Such healthy individuals were said to be *self-actualized*. Therapy concerned itself with the way people in our society try to block off natural parts of themselves to please others, much in the way I spoke of earlier, and therapists attempted to help the patient self-actualize by removing these blockages.

In videotapes of Rogers and Perls at work, they seem to be polar opposites. Rogers is warm, empathic, nonjudgmental, and nonconfrontational—sort of like an ideal grandfather. Perls, on the other hand, is highly confrontational and in-your-face, sharply pointing out right off the bat discrepancies between patients' body language and what they are saying about themselves. Both of them are, however, aiming to help the patient self-actualize. Rogers is providing a warm, accepting environment in which a person is supposed to be able to blossom like a flower and flourish, while Perls wants patients to become hyperaware of and fully experience in their guts what is actually going on inside behind their social masks.

Self-actualization is historically a relatively new and highly Western concept. It is a hallmark of more individualistic cultures and is not even discussed in traditional societies. In traditional societies, people do not care about who an individual would ideally like to be as a person. Members of these societies are supposed to act according to the dictates of their social position and do their duties without complaint. Any members trying to assert themselves outside of accepted norms might be exiled or killed. An illustrative example took place in November 1990 when some women in Saudi Arabia decided as a group to drive cars to stage a protest about women in that country being denied the right to drive. In response, some were arrested or threatened with violence.

The cultural evolution of individuality out of collectivism is brilliantly described by Erich Fromm in his classic book, *Escape from Freedom*.[3] Part of what creates cultural lag is that over history, at least in the West, the forces of individuality have gradually gained strength against the forces of togetherness. The pull by the larger culture for more individualistic behavior butts up against the needs for families to operate by formerly adaptive group rules.

Who in a patient's environment might be working to block the emergence of that person's individuality and interest in breaking old rules? Who are the people whose opinions all Americans care about the most, even if we hate to admit it? The reader would have to know by now that I believe the answer to be the members of a person's family of origin.

In the therapy I administer, helping a patient to self-actualize is clearly my goal. However, my goal is also for patients to be able to freely express their individuality *in the presence* of the people they care about, and to take into consideration the emotional needs of everyone concerned. A family therapist named Murray Bowen termed this type of self-actualization *differentiation of self*. People who are less differentiated chicken out when in the presence of their families and adhere to the family's party line even if they secretly disagree with it vehemently.

Perls wrote about what happens to an individual when important family members have tried to block his or her attempts to self-actualize. He said such patients are left with a sense of having *unfinished business*. In order to help them finish this business, he had patients pretend to talk to a parent or other important attachment figure and to say what they always wanted to say to him or her. This is called the *empty chair* technique because the therapist literally has patients imagine the presence of the significant other sitting in a chair facing them. The patients are supposed to experience what it would be like to say those things.

My question is, why use an empty chair if the parent is still living? Why not try to find a palatable way for the patient to say what he or she needs to say directly to the person? Would that not help the real relationship between the patient and the person with whom the patient has unfinished business? This is actually a trickier question than might appear at first glance.

Should a person who had been, say, sexually abused by a parent try to confront the parent about the abuse and try to reconcile? Perhaps it would be better to completely divorce oneself from such "toxic" parents and never speak to them again, especially if they continue to invalidate their adult child by continuing to deny that the abuse took place. Confronting a parent from a dysfunctional family can also be downright dangerous. Violence or even murder might ensue.

Perhaps it would be best if we all stuck to having one-sided conversations with empty chairs. Alternatively, maybe we should all write down our true feelings in a letter to the person with whom we have unfinished business, and then never mail it. Finding what I believe to be the best answer to this conundrum comes from looking at the fifth major type of psychotherapy, family systems therapy.

FAMILY SYSTEMS THERAPY

As the reader may have gleaned from reading my descriptions, all of the preceding four classes of psychotherapy seem to focus for the most part on what is transpiring inside of the heads of individuals in isolation from their current social environment. However, as I have tried to illustrate, all of them eventually deal with the influence of the patient's family of origin in one way or another.

The last major type of psychotherapy, family systems therapy, looks more explicitly and centrally at the behavior of the kin group as a unit rather than at the individual in isolation. These therapists quickly noticed that the behavior of each member of the family was a major part of what determined the behavior of all the other members of the family. Their ongoing interrelationship was a large determinant of what made each of them who they were.

Family therapists applied systems thinking or *cybernetics* to group behavior. In order for any cohesive group of people to function as a unit that can successfully negotiate environmental challenges, each person must have his or her own role to play, and the whole group has to operate by predictable rules. If instead chaos reigns, the survival of all of the individuals in a group can be threatened. For example, say that a wife has picked up a couple's children from school every day for years without complaint. If the husband comes home one day to unexpectedly find that the wife has willfully left them at school and made no other arrangements for them, this would obviously be a problem. Something bad could happen to small children left alone in a school parking lot after dark.

If in addition to not picking up the kids as usual she suddenly and without warning attacks her husband for being a male chauvinist pig, when she had always in the past acted like she expected him to maintain traditional roles so she would not have to work, this would be highly disorienting to everyone else in the group. The whole family could be easily and irrevocably damaged.

To prevent occurrences such as this, families have developed behavioral feedback loops that stop individuals from acting in unpredictable and potentially harmful ways. When someone in the family tries to break the rules, the rest of the family gangs up on the offender in ways that scream the message "You are wrong; change back." When my patients who have attempted to assert themselves with their families describe this process, they sometimes speak of relatives who have not been involved with them for years suddenly coming out of the woodwork and angrily yelling criticisms like "How can you treat your mother like that?"

I ask the reader to recall the Asch experiments from social psychology described in Chapter Five, in which some subjects denied that short lines were short in order to agree with a group of strangers. Imagine that *everyone you know and care about* comes to you and criticizes you loudly and unmercifully for something you've said. Even if you know that what you said is correct, do you think you would continue to express such a thought?

The feedback loops that keep everyone in line and help the group function in smooth and predictable ways create something called *family homeostasis*. Homeostasis means that a system is kept in equilibrium. This can be best understood by comparing family homeostasis to homeostatic mechanisms in the human body. For instance, if the potassium level in your blood gets too high, your body has compensatory mechanisms to push it back down into the safe range. This is called physiological homeostasis. Family homeostasis works the same way.

Unfortunately, when the culture in which the family operates changes, some of the rules by which the family operates may become seriously outmoded. In that situation, depending on how rigid the rules of the family are, the homeostatic mechanisms that maintain family equilibrium prevent the family from adjusting to new contingencies, and the rules lead the family to function in ways that actually threaten the safety and cohesiveness of the group rather than in ways that help. This is the phenomenon called cultural lag that I described in Chapter Two. As we saw in the case of the societal changes in gender roles, some members of the family may develop individualistic desires to do things that had been up to that point proscribed by the family rules.

Because of a given family's historical experiences and the genetic proclivities of every individual comprising the family, the rules in some families may be more rigidly enforced through homeostatic mechanisms than those in other families. In some families, adjusting the rules to fit new cultural demands, such as allowing for the newly necessary two-career family, is much less of a problem than for others. The family rules also affect the ease with which family members can discuss the rules in a rational way.

The process of communicating about the rules is called *metacommunication*. In many families, such discussions are extremely difficult. Attempts to discuss changing the family rules may be quickly and sometimes viciously invalidated, so people will not even try, even though everyone in the family might be better off if the rules did change, and even though they each might be happier as well.

In families in which metacommunication is rarely attempted, discord between a husband and wife may fester for a long time, because they are unable to discuss their differences in a way that might lead to problem solving. In such cases, according to family systems theory, other family members will either volunteer or be recruited to step in between them to serve as a buffer. This helps to maintain peace within the family, but usually at a big cost in chronic negative feelings. This process is called *triangulation*.

We saw an example of this process in the last chapter with the sister of one of my patients with BPD who would step in to prevent her mother and sister from coming to blows by creating a diversion.

Sometimes the person in the middle seems to ally with one of the warring pair against the other, but he or she may suddenly switch sides at any time and seemingly become an ally of the second person. The shifting alliances are meant to contain any conflicts that may develop between any one individual and the other two that might be triggered by the triangulation process.

The potentially dramatic results of triangulation can commonly be seen in a phenomenon I have witnessed frequently in the mid-South. Middle-aged single women who meet certain parameters come into treatment with me because of chronic dysthymia. They have a career but have had no "luck" at finding a mate or have carried on a long-term relationship with a married man or some other relatively unavailable male who is kept an arm's length. They live within a few blocks of their parents and are constantly "on call" to settle disputes between them. Mother will come over and say things like, "Go talk to your father. I cannot get him to do such and such, but he'll listen to you."

They also have other duties, such as taking care of one of the parents when he or she gets sick so the other parent does not have to, or serving as a companion for one of them when that person needs a break from the chronic tension that exists in the parental relationship. These women may have married siblings who are never called on by the parents to provide any of these services. The parents say things like, "I don't want to bother your sister. She has a family to look after." The unspoken implication is, ". . . and you do not, so it should not be a bother."

The parents do not seem to realize that the prime reason their daughter is single in the first place may be precisely because she thinks it is her job to serve as a buffer between them and that she needs to be available for that purpose, and she believes that she cannot marry if she is to continue to provide this service. Because of what the parents say about their feelings about bothering a married child, she thinks that if she and all of her siblings were married, the parents would be left alone to battle it out with each other. She therefore sacrifices her desire to wed in order to maintain the family homeostasis.

In order to serve this function, she cannot admit to anyone in the family that she is doing what she is doing. If she did, the parents would understandably take offense at her blaming them for the fact that her love life is a disaster rather than blaming her own poor choices or her being "too picky" about potential husbands. After all, they never asked her to buffer their relationship. She would then feel completely invalidated for what she had done for them. Yes, that they did not ask is true, but they seem to need the service and avail themselves of it freely without much thought to the consequences for their daughter.

In order to play a role in a family of origin the purpose of which is to stabilize an unstable parent or a parental dyad, the involved individual creates a false self or persona, mentioned briefly in Chapter Six. In this case, the woman knows down deep that she is keeping men at arm's length through various defensive maneuvers, and she is covertly miserable about it, but she may act as if she is proud of herself for not having gotten "trapped" in a bad relationship. She will not say so unless a therapist knows how to ask the right question, but the bad relationship she is usually thinking about is that between her own parents.

The idea of a false self is something that most family systems theorists reject, because this concept focuses on what is going on inside an individual's head rather than on family process. Even Murray Bowen, founder of one of the three main schools of thought within family systems therapy and whose concept of pseudo-self comes closest to the idea of the false self, probably would have rejected the way I have conceptualized what is taking place.

A problem with systems views is that they sometimes go too far and discount the power of the mind of the individual. Since I have been arguing throughout this book that recent mental health science and clinical practice trends have been moving away from an essential emphasis on family systems behavior, the reader might have assumed that I am in substantial agreement with much of what systems theorists have to say. Actually, in the type of psychotherapy I practice, I work with individuals and not the whole family. Although I do agree with much of family systems theory, some of family systems ideas have once again, unfortunately, turned people's reactions to problematic relationships into mental deficits.

Radical systems therapists share something in common with radical behaviorists: the devaluation of human reasoning, analysis, and thought in favor of thinking that people are totally at the mercy of environmental contingencies. Radical systems people think individuals are completely controlled by cybernetic family feedback loops rather than other types of rewards and punishments, and cannot escape them without some help from forces external to their family system. Some have gone so far as to opine that an individual's belief in his or her own separateness from the system is almost delusional, and they speak of a Zen-like cosmic oneness of the family.

As they train future clinicians to understand feedback loops in families that create dysfunctional family behavior, they invoke the admittedly schematic example of an alcoholic husband and a nagging wife. According to this line of reasoning, a so-called positive feedback loop occurs in which the nagging and drinking behavior of the couple as a dyad together creates a vicious circle that keeps the troublesome pattern going.

The more the alcoholic drinks, the more the nagger nags. The more the nagger nags, the more the drinker drinks, and so forth. The nagger says, "I nag because he drinks," and the drinker says, "I drink because she nags," because each is artificially *punctuating* what is actually a continuous nonstop interaction, and is discounting the effect of his or her own behavior on the other person. The vicious circle keeps this behavior pattern going and going like the Energizer Bunny. When asked how and why it got created in the first place, some of the leaders of family systems theory say they do not know and do not really care. All that matters to them is finding a way to stop it.

For this vicious circle conceptualization to approximate the truth behind such a couple's behavior, we would again have to assume that both the alcoholic and the nagger are insanely stupid and therefore mentally defective. If we assume that these two people are not stupid, we have to assume that they understand on some level what is going on, yet continue in the behavior anyway. A nagger who is not brain dead would have to know after a few rounds of the vicious circle that, at the very least, the husband is using her nagging as an excuse or pretext to continue to drink. He may drink anyway, but her nagging is obviously counterproductive. The drinker tells her so, and his behavior bears it out. The drinker as well would have to know that the nagging about which he is complaining so bitterly is exacerbated by his continuing to drink. If both of these people really want the other person to stop the drinking or nagging, and I do believe this to be the case, then how do we explain the fact that both continue to make the problem worse rather than better?

The problem gets even more complicated if we add in the idea that each member of the couple knows that the other member of the couple is not stupid. How do they explain to themselves why the other person continues to engage in behavior that provokes the very response he or she complains about?

I find that the only way to resolve the paradox created by the apparent blindness of the couple with the idea that people just are not that stupid is to explain the behavior this way: Each member of the couple thinks it's the *other guy* who wants the relationship to continue in its current form despite verbal protestations to the contrary. Each continues his or her behavior *in order* to help or enable the other person to continue with behavior he or she seems so obviously to cherish. The husband, for example, thinks that his wife uses his behavior as a justification for continuing to do what she is already doing—nagging—and that she acts in ways that seem to encourage him to continue to drink. They do not know exactly why the other member of the couple needs to continue to nag or drink, as the case may be.

I believe that the nagger is giving the alcoholic, at great personal sacrifice, a pretext to continue to drink. The fact that he uses this pretext so readily, and continues to provoke the nagging, reinforces her belief that she is correct. The wife would never think in her wildest dreams that her husband continues to drink out of a misguided perception that she really wants him to. If he were to dare say he thought this, she would immediately accuse him of expressing a self-serving and insulting rationalization for his own weakness with respect to alcohol. Likewise, the alcoholic drinks in order to give his wife a pretext to continue to nag, also at great personal cost.

I have actually heard the wives of alcoholics say things like "I can't leave him when he's down like this, but as soon as he stops drinking, I'm out of here!" That sort of statement really will encourage him to stop drinking, don't you think? In couples therapy, couples frequently express the idea that if the relationship ever changes in the way that they both seem to want it to, then it will break up. I used to be shocked by this, as well as by how often I used to hear it. They complain bitterly about each other's behavior, but if it stops, only then will they break up? They will leave if the relationship improves, but stay if it remains awful? The only way this makes sense is if each one secretly believes that it is the other one who needs the relationship to continue in its present form.

I mentioned earlier that I believe both members of this couple really do want the relationship to change, yet at some level they end up making sure that it does not. Since they do whatever they can to maintain the maladaptive relationship, does that not mean they do not want it to change? Am I giving the reader a double message? You have probably forgotten about ambivalence already.

I should have said that they are ambivalent about this change. They hate what they are doing, but they do hang on to it. What I believe is going on here is that each one is enabling the other to maintain a false self. They both had this false self when the couple first met, and it was a major part of what attracted them to each other in the first place. The false self arose from each person's perception of what he or she had to do in order to serve some sort of function within his or her own respective family of origin. They may not understand the subtleties of the concept of sacrificing one-self to help maintain family homeostasis, but that is what they are doing. They also need each other's help in maintaining what is actually a markedly unpleasant set of behaviors. I refer to this as *mutual role function support*.

This whole process is the reason, I believe, that spouses some-times try to subvert the efforts of therapists who focus only on the individual. If a therapist pushes a patient to self-actualize, for exam-ple, the therapist may unknowingly be asking the patient to break a family rule. The spouse knows that the patient needs to obey this rule because breaking it would lead to negative consequences for both the patient and the spouse. For patients, their families of origin might begin to attack them with a vengeance. People tend to fall apart when that happens, and guess who would have to pick up the pieces? Additionally, spouses have a vested interest in the way a patient has always behaved because it helps them to maintain their own false selves.

One helpful thing about the systems perspective is that it predicts that if one person in a family is able to change his or her behavior and make it stick, this will force all the others to change their behavior in some way. Continuing on exactly as before is nearly impossible for the family members unless they exile the person, because they are forced to accommodate to the new behavior. The change one/change all effect in families is sometimes compared to a mobile. If you pull on only one part of a mobile, all of the other parts move.

Of course, a married couple can divorce rather than accommo-date to a spouse's refusal to continue to provide role function sup-port. When this happens, spouses that do not wish to change for fear of upsetting the homeostasis of their own family of origin feel betrayed. They complain about the change even when their spouse has stopped doing something that they themselves may have been complaining about for years.

With parents and children, however, divorce is a bit more com-plicated. Unlike friends or lovers, a parent and child remain emo-tionally connected to each other no matter what they do. If they "divorce" and do not speak to each other, this is called an *emotional cutoff* by systems therapists. For first-degree relatives, systems thera-pists believe that it takes the cooperation of both parties for the cut-off to be maintained. If one person can figure out the right approach to repairing a rupture and persists in the effort, the other will almost invariably respond eventually.

In the section on experiential therapy, I raised the question of whether it is a good idea for an individual to try to resolve

unfinished business with an attachment figure directly with that figure, presuming that person is still living. I pointed out that such
confrontations could be dangerous, and that in some families any
attempt to metacommunicate about family rules is met with instant
invalidation. Nonetheless, I have found that finding a way to stop
the parents or other primary attachment figures from advertently or
inadvertently reinforcing those old limbic system fear tracts is the
quickest way to help people learn to override them and to make
needed changes. The question is not whether they should approach
the parents and metacommunicate, but how it should be done.
Doing it badly is indeed worse than not doing it at all.

In the next and final chapter, I will give my own ideas about
ways to integrate the different schools of psychotherapy and biological psychiatry as well as to restore the field's emphasis on helping
people cope better with their problematic relationships instead of
merely treating the psychological symptoms that result from them.

10

Integration

In the summer of 1983, psychologists Paul Wachtel, Marvin Goldfried, George Striker, Barry Wolfe, Jeanne Phillips, and psychiatrist Lee Birk began an association that led to the founding of an academic group dedicated to the search for common ground among psychodynamic and cognitive-behavioral therapists. Gradually, academic therapists from most of the other major schools of thought were attracted to the group. The group was named the Society for the Exploration of Psychotherapy Integration (SEPI). They began to have annual meetings and their own journal.

The group's rather cumbersome name stemmed from the fact that the founders of the group were fearful that if they actually proposed a completely integrated model, then they would be in danger of being just one more school—the "integrated" school. They feared that this development would lead to the exclusion from the group of both loyal adherents to the existing schools and anyone with a new idea that did not seem to fit in with the new model. Hence they decided to only "explore" ideas that were conducive to finding areas of agreement between the schools.

Since the organization consisted mostly of nonmedical therapists, psychiatric ideas about the underlying biology of human mental processes were at first not part of the mix of ideas considered by the group. Later, some newer developments in neurobiology were seen by some group members as actually supporting much of what psychotherapists had been saying. Psychiatrists in the group, along with some psychologists, began to bring these additional viewpoints into SEPI.

Another important development in the search for common ground took place in 1985. The Milton Erickson Foundation in Phoenix, Arizona, invited all of the leading thinkers of the various schools of psychotherapy who were still living to a conference. Erickson was an expert in the subtle uses of hypnosis, and many of his ideas helped to inspire the therapeutic techniques used by family systems therapists. The conference was called the Evolution of Psychotherapy, and therapists from all over the country came to watch their heroes in action.

This was a milestone in psychotherapy integration because the conference was structured in a way that allowed the leaders of various schools to comment on the ideas of the other schools. The conference was so successful that it was repeated in 1990. By then, some of the therapy innovators from the first conference had already passed away, but new leaders took their place.

THE TOWER OF PSYCHOBABBLE REVISITED

As a psychiatry resident in the mid-1970s, I had been so turned off by all the competing voices in the different psychotherapy schools that I decided against being a therapist. I felt, as did many physicians, that psychotherapy was unscientific. I became a biological psychiatrist, and I took a hospital job treating the chronically and persistently mentally ill. This period in my life lasted about two years. Before the two years were up, I had come to the conclusion that illnesses like schizophrenia were neurological rather than psychological disorders. I became bored. I began to feel like I was nothing more than a Haldol salesman. (Haldol was the leading antipsychotic medication at that time.) When I made the jump to private practice in 1979, I decided to give psychotherapy another look.

I was strongly influenced by a psychologist colleague, the late Michael Braver. He introduced me to two areas of thought to which I had not been exposed. The first was scientific philosophy. He gave me Kuhn's classic work, *The Structure of Scientific Revolutions*, from which the infamous phrase "paradigm shift" was introduced into the lexicon. This book explains why so many competing viewpoints exist in a young science like psychotherapy. Michael also introduced me to family systems thinking.

Whenever a patient would cancel an appointment at the last minute or not show, I would grab a book about one or the other of the different schools of psychotherapy and read voraciously. I would try out the various interventions that the books suggested on my patients to see what sort of reactions I would get and if the interventions seemed to work as well as the books described. Although many of these therapeutic interventions proved very useful at times, they often did not work as advertised.

The last category of psychotherapy schools I initiated reading about was family systems therapy, and the last subschool of family therapy I came across was that of Bowen.[1] His work was an eye opener, and I was blown away. I felt that he actually had integrated a lot of the ideas I had read about from other schools in a novel and extremely powerful way. His followers, of course, thought nothing of the sort. They insisted that what they were saying had absolutely nothing in common with the other schools, and they seemed to be as dogmatic as anyone.

I had also by then read a fair amount of material from other disciplines like evolutionary biology. I read *Escape from Freedom* about the emergence of individuality from collectivism. I decided that I wanted to try my hand at integrating all the ideas and began to write a book just for fun. I had no publisher and I did not send out sample chapters to get a publishing contract. When I finally finished it, I sent the whole manuscript to fourteen publishers of psychotherapy books, and I was lucky enough to get accepted by one of them.

During the writing of the book, I attended the Evolution of Psychotherapy Conference. It was thrilling. Watching the founding fathers like Rogers, Bowen, Salvador Minuchin, Ellis, Joseph Wolpe, and others interact, I began to feel more strongly about the ideas that I had been coming up with. The meeting also inspired a few new ideas. Still, I was bedeviled by one paradox: Why would smart people continue to engage in the same seemingly counterproductive behavior over and over again with the same results? Every time I thought I had figured out the answer, my mind seemed to lose its grasp of the idea. Clearly, what I was attempting to understand ran counter to my normal way of thinking. In fact, the answer ran counter to normal intuition; it was *counterintuitive*. This may be why so many therapists miss it.

WHY ARE PATIENTS NOT DOING THE OBVIOUS?

With my patients, I somehow stumbled on a version of a therapeutic question that had, unbeknownst to me, first been proposed by Adler, one of the three founding fathers of psychodynamic psychotherapy. I asked my patients why they were not employing the obvious solutions to their problems. When a therapist does that, the first answer he or she gets is one described by Eric Berne, founder of a psychotherapy school called transactional analysis.[2] In essence, the answer goes something like "Yes, I could do that *but* . . ." followed by some lame excuse for why they cannot do that. This is known as the game of *Why Don't You—Yes But*.

I decided I would play my own version of the game, which I called *Why I Can't—Yes But*. Every time I heard a yes-but answer to my original question, I would counter with "Yes, but you could handle that obstacle by doing [such and such]." This solution would also be yes-butted by the patient with another lame excuse, for which I would provide another obvious solution.

For example, one adult female could not seem to hold a job and always seemed to end up going back home to live with and depend upon on her abusive father and inadequate mother. I knew other relatives also lived in the home, but I had no clue as to their significance. The woman was bright and had made it to the upper echelons of a sport that she liked to play, so I knew she was highly capable of holding a job. Every time she offered an excuse such as "I'm no good in school so I can't learn new skills," I would counter with my own yes-but. I went through a seemingly endless array of lame excuses in this manner, until finally she said, "If I'm not at the house, my father molests my niece."

This answer caught me completely off guard. He does *what*? I had trouble coming up with a new yes-but of my own. Finally I said, "Have you thought about reporting him to child protective services?" She replied, "Of course, but if I did that my mother would end up on the street because she cannot support herself, and she would blame me."

Well, lessee. She could handle that obstacle to holding a job by . . . by . . . by . . . er, how exactly could she handle that problem? I had no answer. She could write her mother off, I suppose, but since when is caring about the survival of family members a bad thing? This was a really devilish conundrum. I also wondered why she had not told me about this in the first place. That was the moment that I was first confronted by evidence that family members may be acting for altruistic motives rather than selfish ones, and that family problems might be incredibly difficult to solve.

Her response also provided an important clue to the answer to my conundrum about the repetition compulsion. Individuals do the same things over and over because it solves a problem in the best way they know how and because other family members seem to need them to continue to act the way they do. I had read about the idea that individuals sacrifice themselves for the seeming good of their families in a book by Mara Selvini-Palazzoli,[3] but I really did not get it. Since then, other writers like Lorna Benjamin have made similar discoveries. She said, "Every pathology is a gift of love."[4]

I then found a way to shorten the endless yes-butting process to more quickly get to the altruistic motive behind self-destructive behavior. I had learned of Adler's actual version of the question and began asking a version closer to the original: "What if I had a magic wand and could make this problem go away? What would be the downside of that?" A few patients were able to quickly give the altruistic answer.

For example, one of my residents treated a patient who constantly tortured herself with catastrophic predictions in her thinking of worst-case scenarios, even when her life was going well. She would refuse lucrative promotions at work because of these self-scaring thoughts. When my resident asked, "What would happen if you were able to stop doing that?" she replied without hesitation, "My father would not know what to do with himself, and he would stop sending me money."

Most of the time, however, in response to the Adlerian question, patients respond in less forthcoming ways. They may stare blankly and say, "I don't know." If the therapist gets quiet, encourages the patient to free-associate, and listens without interruption, the answer gradually comes out over the next few sessions. Some patients say, "I would just find some other way to screw up my life." By this they mean they would come up with some different behavioral strategy that would leave their lives in pretty much the same shape as it already is. In this situation, I counter with, "Suppose my magic wand prevented you from screwing things up by any means? What would be the downside of that happening?"

Another common response is "I cannot even picture that situation in my head." This is a seemingly bizarre thing to say. People can imagine just about anything, no matter how impossible. I can picture in my mind flapping my arms and flying. What do the patients mean, they cannot imagine something? I counter this answer with "Well, that must mean that the downside, whatever it is, is so upsetting that you are afraid to even think about it. What might that downside be?" This question then often leads to the answer that if the problem were solved, patients would become even more self-destructive than before. They might start cutting themselves more, for example. I counter again with "Well, again that must mean that you would be really upset about something. What do you think that something is?"

In addition to the Adlerian questions, I also started to ask patients questions like "What does your mother say about your problem?" If a patient is engaged in self-destructive repetitive patterns with a spouse, I might even ask, "What does your father-in-law say about this argument you two have been having?" In response to these questions, I started to hear the most amazing things—things I had never heard said by patients in therapy before I started to ask the right questions. This is a case of "don't ask-don't tell." If the therapist does not ask, the patient does not tell.

ELIMINATING THE MIDDLE MAN

The next obvious major piece of the puzzle for me was finding the answer to the question: Now that you know what is happening with the patient and a bit about why, what can you do about it? I found my answer in a criticism of the work of Bowen by a SEPI member named Daniel Wile.[5] Bowen was the only family systems theorist who worked with individuals. He was the one who started using genograms to trace the evolution of dysfunctional family relationship patterns.

His therapy was primarily educational in nature. He would use what Wile called nonmanipulative means such as education, logic, and collaboration to help his patients understand their family dynamics and their own role within those dynamics. He would then coach his patients to go back to their families of origin to change the family rules.

If they were successful, these changes would generalize or carry over to their other intimate relationships, far more than a change in the transference relationship with a psychodynamic therapist generalizes to other relationships. I believe this is true because, as I have argued, those early limbic system fear tracks are reinforced more powerfully by primary attachment figures than by anything or anyone else. These tracks are what create mental schemas or models for how to behave in all social contexts in which the individual travels. Why should a therapist recreate the relationship with the parents through the generation of transference when the original triggers to the problem behavior are still alive? My motto became "eliminate the middle man."

Wile's criticism of Bowen was that when Bowen coached his patients on how to change the rules with their families, he taught them to use the manipulative techniques that are used by the other family systems schools, such as reverse psychology, double binds, and other strategic maneuvers. Why did he not coach his patients to use the same techniques with their families that he used with his patients? Why did he teach them to be *strategic* family therapists with their families and not Bowen family therapists?

At the Evolution of Psychotherapy Conference, I asked Carl Whitaker, another family systems pioneer, what he thought of Bowen's work. He replied rather cryptically that he thought Bowen must have been a very lonely guy. Several weeks went by before I figured out what he might have meant. When Bowen used strategic techniques on his own family of origin, as he described in a paper he published, he essentially distanced himself from them. He extricated himself from his role in the family drama and from the family itself, rather than changing the family drama for the better while remaining a part of it. With no close family, Whitaker must have reasoned, Bowen must have been lonely.

In my practice and eventually in my book, I began to modify Bowen's techniques to train my patients to become Bowen therapists with their families of origin. To do so, the patient and I would have to figure out and practice ways to get past the family members' rather formidable defenses and other family homeostatic mechanisms, so as to allow for rational discussion of the origins and nature of the family rules and if following them remained a good idea. For this metacommunicative strategy to be successful, the patient had to learn empathy for all members of the family no matter how heinous some of their behavior had been.

Empathy means trying to understand why the others felt they needed to act like they did without condoning obviously bad behavior such as child abuse. Condoning it as well as understanding it would be sympathy rather than empathy. Sympathy in this situation is in fact incompatible with empathy. If an adult child were to say to a formerly abusive parent, "What you did was OK," the parent would know the child was not being sincere. Parents know this because they are not stupid. Despite any denial or protestations to the contrary, everyone knows that child abuse is an evil thing that no one in his or her right mind would ever welcome. Being insincere is never empathic.

Empathy for misbehaving relatives is not always easy to muster, even for a therapist. How can anyone be warm and understanding with someone who has committed despicable acts? Empathic with a child molester? You have got to be kidding, right? No. The therapist's job is to help the patient find something redeeming about everyone in his or her family. The motive may not justify the means, but it does count for something. As Albert Ellis pointed out, people are not synonymous with their actions. When the therapist and patient construct the genogram, it usually puts the parents' bad behavior in a whole new light.

Finding empathy is essential for effective metacommunication. Anything that smacks of blaming, attacking, or other similar actions

or verbalizations will immediate cause the object to go into fight-
or-flight mode. If that happens during an attempt by an adult child
to metacommunicate with a parent, the parent will refuse to discuss
anything rationally, continue to exhibit distancing or invalidating
behavior, or counterattack viciously without mercy.

I discovered that for metacommunication in dysfunctional families, generic assertiveness techniques do not work because of the
high levels of family defensiveness and the rigid homeostatic rules.
The approach to any given family member has to be individually
tailored to his or her sensitivities and concerns. Furthermore, to prevent the rest of the family ganging up on my patients to invalidate
their attempts to bring up sensitive family issues, the relatives have
to be approached one at a time. Before doing that, strategies for
stopping other family members from interfering, known as *detrian-
gulating strategies*, have to be devised.

As I mentioned earlier in this book, patients have proven to be
masters at predicting the responses of targeted family members to
various interventions. What I would do to find out the best way to
approach a family member was to have patients play-act the family
member. I used role-playing in this manner so I could see what they
were up against. I would try out various strategies to see what
might work the best and to predict the problems and defenses that
the targeted family member might use in response. The patient and
I would work together until we came up with something that the
patient thought might work. We would then trade places and
I would play the targeted family member and allow the patient to
practice the strategy we had worked out.

The resulting treatment paradigm as well as the theory behind
it, which I called *unified therapy*, became the subject of my first book
in the field and a major part of my life's work. As I mentioned earlier in this volume, seeing formerly estranged or warring family
members reconcile is one of the most moving and fulfilling experiences a therapist can have.

CONSILIENCE

After my book came out, I learned of the existence of SEPI and
joined. The first meeting I attended was a wonderful experience.
I enjoyed the company of people who had the same interests as
mine. As the years passed, however, I gradually began to feel that
the meetings were becoming a little stale. I became somewhat impa-
tient with the insistence of the group's leaders on "exploring" rather
than actually doing psychotherapy integration. While members

sometimes emphasized ideas from other disciplines like social psychology, sociology, history, linguistics, and neurobiology, I thought these ideas needed to be more central to attempts at integration.

From time to time other voices echoed my thoughts. Most notably, Bernard Beitman, chairman of psychiatry at the University of Missouri in Columbia, wrote an article that begged the group to "stop exploring." More recently, fellow traveler Jeffrey Magnavita also began to push for moves toward unifying the different theories. The patron saint of the unification movement is sociobiologist E. O. Wilson, author of the book *Consilience*,[6] whose theme is that various sources of knowledge must and will eventually come together.

I continue to be active in SEPI as associate editor of their journal, the *Journal of Psychotherapy Integration*. I believe that efforts at integrating ideas from many academic disciplines will continue and will be the wave of the future, finally winning out over the forces of reductionism or looking at human functioning from a far too narrow perspective like neurotransmitter functioning.

Although I have been highly critical of some of the limitations of the existing schools of psychotherapy as well as the prescribing practices of many so-called biological psychiatrists, I want to reiterate something I wrote in the introduction. Many psychiatrists, psychologists, clinical social workers, and marriage and family therapists continue to do outstanding work. Help for the most difficult emotional problems is available. Many therapists and psychiatrists take the time to get to the bottom of their clients' problems and their unhappiness and offer specific interventions to solve problems. They do not just tell them to cover up their bad feelings with medication or merely provide a shoulder for them to cry on.

However, finding a good clinician is not always easy, so I would like to offer a few suggestions. Unfortunately, outside of getting a recommendation from a trusted source, one cannot usually tell how good a clinician is before entering his or her consulting room. In the next two sections, I will list some of the ways a knowledgeable consumer of mental health services can tell whether he or she is getting a good evaluation and good treatment. I will start with suggestions for appraising recommendations from psychiatrists and other doctors about the use of psychiatrically active medication.

FINDING A GOOD PSYCHOPHARMACOLOGIST: GOOD AND BAD SIGNS

The most telltale sign that differentiates good versus bad medication management is the time the physician takes to take your history as well as how complete the history is. A complete initial psychiatric history takes at the very minimum 45 minutes to an hour, depending on the complexity of your clinical condition. Those doctors who rely mostly on symptom checklists, without a clear understanding of the person behind the symptom and his or her psychosocial environment, are the mostly likely to be dupes of the medical-industrial shenanigans described in Chapters Four and Six.

The elements of a complete psychiatric history were described in Chapter Seven. The social history is the part of the history that is most often left out in history taking nowadays, but a psychiatrist cannot really know the diagnostic significance of any symptom without this background information.

Particularly if you have chronic mood or anxiety problems, questions that should be asked of you include: How often do the symptoms occur? How long do they last? Are there any things or events in your environment or personal relationships that trigger them? Does anything make them go away? If you experience several symptoms, do they all come at the same time? Do they come and go depending on what is happening to you at the time, or do they stay regardless of what is happening in your life? Do you have periods in between episodes during which you feel essentially all right?

I have spent considerable time in this volume discussing the vicissitudes of the diagnosis of bipolar disorder. If your doctor tells you that you have this disorder, you need to carefully assess how he or she came to that conclusion. Did the doctor ask all of the above questions? An additional question the doctor should have asked is whether you have a family history of bipolar disorder.

Bipolar disorder is highly genetic, so if you do not have a family history of it, the odds that you have it go down considerably. You do have to keep in mind that sometimes families are very secretive about old Aunt Bessie who was hospitalized or who committed suicide, so you may not really know for certain if you have a family history of the disorder. You also may be acquainted with only your mother's or your father's side of the family, and therefore you may not know for this reason. Last, if you are adopted, you of course may not know the extended family history of your biological parents.

If you truly have episodes of bipolar mania or depression, the way that you feel in the midst of an episode should be markedly different from the way you feel when you are not. In mania, people do things they would never even dream of doing in the euthymic state, such as picking up strangers and having unprotected sex. Psychotic symptoms such as grandiose delusions that may be present during an episode, always indicative of a serious mental disorder, should disappear completely after the episode clears.

Although stress can trigger a manic or a major depressive episode, once the symptoms take hold they should take on a life of their own. No matter what happens environmentally, the severity of the symptoms does not change markedly over a short period of time. During a clear-cut major depressive episode, for example, a person could literally win the lottery and hardly crack a smile. The depressed state should last at least two weeks straight, and symptoms should be experienced nearly all day nearly every day.

The severity of the symptoms may change slightly at different times during this stretch, but not drastically, and the individual should almost constantly be aware of being depressed. If you are able to go out with your friends and temporarily completely forget about how bad you are feeling, you may have some other form of depression.

Patients in the midst of an acute manic state should probably be first treated in a hospital environment, because they are likely to be highly unreliable about taking medication. The best treatment for acute mania in the hospital setting is lithium plus an antipsychotic medication. If a manic patient has been unresponsive to lithium in the past, Depakote is a reasonable alternative. The antipsychotic medication is used initially because so-called mood stabilizers like lithium usually take two weeks to work, while the antipsychotic medications work much more quickly.

Depakote or Tegretol can be substituted for lithium if the patient does not tolerate it. After the episode clears and the patient is out of the hospital and stable for a few weeks, the antipsychotic medications should be tapered off so that only one drug is being used. Often doctors do not do this and continue the antipsychotic medication needlessly. Two drugs are only necessary in a minority of truly bipolar patients for mania prevention.

For patients who are not acutely ill and are therefore appropriate for outpatient treatment, the doctor should be able to make a good case for a diagnosis of bipolar disorder. You should have had clear-cut and well-demarcated "high" periods in the past. The doctor should then discuss several different treatment options with you. I would be especially concerned if the doctor does not mention lithium as the best option, or if he or she seems determined to start you on an atypical antipsychotic or Lamictal right off the bat.

If you are taking lithium, your blood levels of the drug need to be checked every month until stable, and then every two to three months. True bipolar disorder requires that you stay on the medication indefinitely. The reason is that when patients are becoming manic, unlike when they are becoming depressed, they seldom realize it before it is too late. By then they can do significant damage to their relationships, careers, financial status, and reputation.

Whenever a psychiatrist starts you on any medication, he or she should ask you if you have any concerns about taking psychiatric medications, and discuss these concerns with you. Some patients are worried that taking psychiatric medications means they are weak or that they are insufficiently pious in practicing their religion. Others worry that they might become dependent on the medication or that they would be using medication as a crutch. The doctor should also inquire if you have friends, relatives, or fellow members of a twelve-step program for addiction who might give you a hard time about taking medications, and suggest ways to handle this.

For the less severe chronic type of depression such as that which characterizes dysthymia, and for almost any chronic anxiety disorder such as generalized anxiety or panic disorder, a good psychiatrist should in most instances recommend psychotherapy along with medication. Psychiatrists who are not themselves therapists should offer you the names of good psychologists or other nonmedical therapists and strongly recommend that you make an appointment with them in addition to making a follow-up appointment with the psychiatrist to assess your response to the medication. This is especially important if you cannot identify clear triggers to your symptoms, if the symptoms are accompanied by repetitive self-destructive or self-defeating behavior patterns, or if you are experiencing chronic and overt family discord.

For almost all psychiatric diagnoses, but especially with mood and anxiety disorders, good psychiatric follow-up is essential. Often when internists or family doctors prescribe antidepressants, they do not make a follow-up appointment. They assume that if they do not hear from a patient, the patient must be doing all right. This is about as far from my experience as one could get.

Often patients do not respond to the first agent prescribed at the lowest possible dosage; they may have severe side effects yet continue to take the medication, or they sometimes decide not to take it at all because of the side effects. They may not call the doctor back to inform him or her of these developments, either because of a lack of initiative caused by depression or because they do not want to be a bother to the doctor. You should be seen at least every three weeks until your mood returns to its baseline state, or more often if suicidality is an issue.

Good psychiatric follow-up is not just asking about a few symptoms, writing a prescription, and sending you on your merry way.

According to the APA official practice guidelines for major depression,[7] psychiatric management includes evaluating the safety of the patients and others, evaluating the level of the patients' functional impairments, establishing and maintaining a good relationship with patients, providing education about patients' illness to patients and their families, enhancing compliance with treatment, and working with patients to address early signs of relapse.

This list only applies to the type of visit referred to as "medication management." Psychotherapy is an additional consideration. If you have been stable on your medications for a while, these activities may only take a few minutes, but otherwise, these services cannot be adequately completed in a seven-minute follow-up appointment.

After your mental state returns to baseline, you should still be seen by your doctor in person every two to four months while you are on active psychiatric medication. If you have just had your first or second clear-cut episode of major depression, the doctor should discuss tapering off an antidepressant after six months to a year to see if you still need it. Unfortunately, a doctor has no way of knowing if you do except through the use of trial and error. Antidepressants do work to prevent future episodes, but some people may not have another one for years, at which time the antidepressant that worked previously can be restarted. In the meantime, you can save yourself the time, expense, and side effects of the medication.

Some patients do not care about these latter considerations and do not want to risk ever experiencing their symptoms again. They may elect to stay on antidepressants prophylactically. A decision about staying on these medications indefinitely should be your call. Paradoxically, patients with dysthymia who do respond to antidepressants often need to stay on medication for much longer periods of time than patients with clear-cut major depression, and they are more likely to also require psychotherapy so they can eventually get off the drugs. Good evidence also exists that good psychotherapy can help to reduce the life stresses that are likely to precipitate future major depressive episodes, and thereby reduce the frequency of recurrences.

FINDING A GOOD THERAPIST

Asking about the training and theoretical orientation of a potential therapist is a good first step, but often not particularly telling. Therapists within any theoretical school can be either good therapists or bad therapists. Also, most therapists today have one "home" school with which they are most familiar but liberally borrow ideas and treatment techniques from two or three other schools.

In other words, most therapists are eclectic, and that is a good thing, unless they use techniques indiscriminately and incoherently in ways that create confusion rather than enlightenment.

Psychiatrists, psychologists, clinical social workers, and marriage and family therapists can all be effective therapists, just as many of them can be ineffective. They all may subscribe to any of the different psychotherapy schools. Psychiatrists who do therapy have, as I have indicated, been decreasing in number. The ones who continue to do therapy can also handle your medication needs at the same time, as well as understand and help you with any problematic interactions between your psychological and medical conditions that you may have. Split treatment is workable but is less cost efficient.

Good therapists will generally be empathic, nonjudgmental, and personable without being too familiar. They will not be afraid to ask you difficult questions that might upset you or make you cry, nor will they be completely insensitive to how difficult opening up may be for you. They will not be threatened if you question their credentials or if you express interest in getting more than one opinion about your problem. If you experience a negative reaction to something they do or say, they should be open and nondefensive about discussing your thoughts and feelings about it. Of course, they will never under any circumstances try to have a relationship with you of any kind outside the consulting room, nor a relationship other than that between a client and a therapist while inside the office.

Good therapists will, after they evaluate you, offer you some sort of verbal treatment contract that specifies, with your agreement, what behaviors or bad feeling states you are there to work on and change. Treatment goals in the contract should be specific and measurable, so that you will know if and when the therapy has been successful and should therefore discontinue sessions. These goals may be changed later in therapy if new information comes to light, although only with your agreement.

Although therapists may not be able to be specific about how exactly they will approach your problem until they get to know you much better, the treatment contract should also inform you in general about what you are expected to do during the early therapy sessions, and something about what the therapist will do in response. The therapist should address any concerns you have about treatment, and also inquire about any potential behavior that you might engage in that would interfere either with the process of therapy or with a successful outcome.

A therapist is not supposed to be just a paid friend who asks you about how your week went, allows you to ventilate feelings, and provides you with a shoulder to cry on. If that is all that the therapist is doing for a significant period of time, then you should probably look for another one. Although personal growth per se is not an invalid treatment goal if you want to pay for that out of your own pocket, I personally do not believe that medical insurance should pay for a treatment in which that is the only goal. Most of the time, psychotherapy treatment should address and try to resolve specific problems. It is designed to do two things: find out what is creating the problems, and then figure out how you can fix them.

In any good therapy, you should learn something. You should gain insight into yourself and your significant others, and learn new behavioral strategies and coping skills that can be used to improve both your situation and the way you feel. I never cease to be amazed at the number of times I have asked patients what they learned from a previous therapist, and in response they stare back at me blankly as if to say, "You mean I was supposed to learn something?" Often they cannot seem to remember what it is they were working on in therapy or if it had anything to do with the complaint they came to me with.

One aspect of a therapist's behavior that you should be wary of is the use of what has been called "accusatory interpretations." In some types of psychodynamic therapy, patients are believed to behave the way they do because they have suffered from a case of arrested development and are therefore functioning at the level of a two-year-old. No matter how the therapist dresses it up, that kind of statement is an insult. In my opinion it just is not true.

For certain psychiatric problems, one or two types of psycho-therapy treatment interventions have been shown to be more effective that the others, but for many problems no clear evidence exists that one school is superior to another. In most cases of a simple, single, isolated psychological symptom, going to a psychodynamically oriented therapist would be a waste of time. You should in that case seek a cognitive behavioral therapist. For example, if you have a public speaking phobia that was never an issue in the past because you never had to speak publicly, but due to a promotion you suddenly need to give oral presentations to do your job, short-term treatment with a CBT therapist would in most instances help you get over your fears.

Patients who are not very disturbed can usually benefit from just about any standard type of psychotherapy in which the therapist is empathic and helps them to think about their problems consistently in a new way that makes sense to them. Obviously, just like with any medical condition, the more severe a psychiatric problem is, the worse the prognosis, no matter what sort of treatment is given. Unlike problematic and highly distressing reactions to one-of-a-kind environmental situations such as an unexpected loss of a loved one, chronic ongoing problems usually require longer-term therapy.

An old joke among therapists is that the best candidate for all types of psychotherapy is a YAVIS. That acronym stands for young, attractive, verbal, intelligent, and successful. One might ask why such people would ever even need therapy, although they too can suffer from significant emotional distress and need help. Surely, the YAVIS is the best candidate for brief rather than long-term therapy.

When it comes to treatment for chronic dysthymia or anxiety symptoms with unclear triggers, chronic repetitive self-defeating or self-destructive behavior patterns, severe family discord, multiple complex psychiatric complaints, or severe personality disorders, longer-term treatment is probably going to be more beneficial than short-term treatment. As I mentioned, the interventions used by many schools of treatment start to look a lot more alike when it comes to these cases.

For these types of problems, in this book I have been advocating for the psychotherapy schools that pay particular attention to ongoing interpersonal and family relationship patterns and that help you to change the patterns with the real live people with whom you are involved. Unfortunately, many of the treatment strategies that specifically address family problems in this manner are not widely practiced, and finding a good therapist who does this sort of work may take time and effort.

In addition to my own treatment paradigm called "unified therapy," I would recommend therapists who are familiar with techniques from *Bowen family systems therapy*,[8] Lorna Benjamin's *interpersonal reconstructive therapy*,[9] Paul Wachtel's *relational therapy*,[10] Jeffrey Magnavita's *personality-guided relational psychotherapy*,[11] Anthony Ryle's *cognitive-analytic therapy*,[12] or Jeffrey Young's *schema therapy*.[13]

In the last sections of the book, I would like to address those readers who have parents or adult children from whom they are either estranged or with whom they have a consistently hostile, unpleasant, or unsettling relationship.

RECONCILIATION

When I first bring up the idea of repairing broken family-of-origin relationships with my patients who come from dysfunctional or abusive families, I am often told by them that they would really prefer to have no relationship with their families at all. Nonetheless, they have been unable to extricate or divorce themselves from parents or adult children who are driving them insane. I cannot count the times I have heard the statement "I love them to death, but I just cannot be around them." That bit about loving them to death always fascinated me. Could the phrase betray all the hidden rage they feel while at the same time betraying their fervent desire to remain connected?

As I have argued, even for patients who are estranged from family members, the effects of their past relationships on them continue to be profound. Some are afraid to have children because they are afraid they might mistreat them. This is a valid concern. Although nothing is written in stone, attachment studies have shown that the best predictor for how new parents will relate to their children is the nature of their attachment to their own parents.

I must garner all my powers of persuasion to convince patients that attempting to reconcile with difficult parents or difficult adult children is a good idea. While it is often true that they can hardly stand to be around problematic relatives now with the relationships in their present form, I tell them that they *would* want a relationship if the relationship were not so frequently unbearable. When reconciliation and new interpersonal understanding take place between family members, the benefits are immeasurable.

I am also frequently told by patients that their parents or their adult children are the most difficult people in the world, and that getting them to change their obnoxious behavior and listen to reason is an impossible task. They add that no one could conceivably be worse than their family. If I just knew these people, I would see that. After having invited many family members in for conjoint questions, I can certainly empathize with those sentiments.

However, after having been doing this work for over thirty years, I can assure them that I have in fact seen families who act worse than theirs. In some cases, I have seen much worse. I tell them that I am certain that a connection between parents and their children can almost always be found that can be exploited for purposes of reconciliation, and that a way can be found to get past the defenses of the other family members and improve the relationship between the patient and the significant other.

The patients are also told that I am not asking them to "fix" their significant others or to change them in a fundamental way. I agree that they do not have the power to do that, nor is that their job. What they do have the power to do is change *their relationship* with those people. Because of the mobile effect posited by family systems theory, if they change their approach to another family member, that family member is forced to change his or her behavior toward them. The family member might try various ruses to get the patient to back off, but those behavioral strategies can also be countered. Where there is a will, there is a way. The family members may or may not continue to act the same way with the rest of the world, but their relationship with the patient will change.

Ironically, most of the patients' problematic behavior stems from their attempt to fix other family members in the first place. Their attempts have backfired precisely because they seldom have the power to directly fix another person, and their behavior instead precludes the one activity that might stand a chance: metacommunication about family dynamics. Problems need to be discussed, not acted out, in order to be solved. I add that if anything is going to help the targeted family members change their general problem behavior, metacommunication about the family dynamics stands the best chance of doing so. Of course, I can offer no guarantees that such a transformation will take place. Happily, it sometimes does.

When discussions regarding ongoing family problems are avoided, the hidden reason is often that the family members are afraid of hurting each other's feelings. I refer to this as a *protection racket*. In spite of a patient's insistence that other family members need to suffer because of their misdeeds, the forces of kin selection operate so that the family members' biggest fear is often making an important relative feel bad. In addition to the protection racket preventing a problem from being discussed in a way through which it might actually be solved, it also communicates the message "You are such a weak person that you cannot tolerate any unpleasant feelings." Paradoxically, receiving this message from loved ones makes individuals feel weak and makes them more likely to act as if they truly cannot tolerate a frank discussion.

Even some therapists avoid the use of anxiety-provoking discussions with patients when they are called for. When a patient then overreacts anyway in response, the therapist feels justified for having been restrained, not realizing that his or her attitude about the strength of the patient helped induce the patient to overreact. After all, therapists are supposed to be experts on human emotions. If they think a patient is weak, who is the patient to argue?

DO YOU NEED A THERAPIST?

In most cases, I would not recommend that people who come from violent, severely abusive, or extremely discordant families try to reconcile with other family members without the help of a therapist. As I mentioned, attempting to do so and doing it badly is far worse than never trying to do it at all. Although some people may naturally be very good at researching their genogram to try to understand and empathize with their parents, and then finding ways to gently get past family resistances in order to metacommunicate in a way that successfully changes problematic patterns, most are not.

The majority of people from such families have a great deal of trouble coming up with a successful strategy on their own and then keeping their cool long enough to complete it. To be successful, individuals often have to tackle family members' multiple levels of denial one after the other, as well as weather attacks from well-meaning relatives or even family friends or clergymen. They must be prepared for vicious counterattacks, guilt trips, feigned outrage, and a host of other maneuvers. If this were an easy task, they probably would have done it years ago. Usually the help of an expert who has more knowledge about the reasons for odd human behavior and how to counter it is needed.

Some therapists who do this kind of work make what I consider to be two basic mistakes that can lead to a bad outcome. The first is using what I refer to as an *ambush interview*. I borrow this phrase from the television newsmagazine *Sixty Minutes*, in which it is used to describe a reporter who appears at an evildoer's house unexpectedly with a TV crew and confronts him with the charges against him. The second error is the related problem of not allowing formerly abusive parents to save face.

Bringing unsuspecting family members to a session with the patient and then revealing or bringing up for the first time some past misbehavior of a family member that the patient has told the therapist about is hazardous and counterproductive. In this situation, the family members feel cornered as well as humiliated, and their reactions are not pretty. In fact, springing this on a family can scuttle future attempts by the patient to metacommunicate and may also lead to a malpractice suit against the therapist.

One patient of mine had this experience with a former therapist. The therapist brought the family into a session and told the parents for the first time that their son, the patient's brother, had molested her when the siblings were both teenagers. By the time the session was over, the parents had convinced the therapist that the patient was exaggerating and that nothing untoward had happened. They all agreed, except for the patient of course, that what had happened was nothing more than innocent horseplay.

Needless to say, the patient quit therapy with the former therapist and did not see another one for years. Furthermore, the session
led to a complete emotional cutoff between the patient and the
parents that lasted for just as many years. By the time she came to
me, she literally did not know if they were alive or dead. I was completely unsuccessful at convincing her of the wisdom of trying to
reconnect with them. Her reluctance was understandable.

Some therapists also advise their patients to take legal action
against abusive parents or go public with their accusations. My
advice is that if a therapist suggests that you do that, find another
therapist. Publicly humiliating your relatives is no way to try to
make peace with them. Both public revelations and ambush interviews do not allow the parents to save face.

Some popular authors who write self-help books that advise
individuals who were sexually abused as children about how to discuss the issue with the abuser say that a parent who has done such
awful things has forfeited the right to save face. I completely disagree. The object of discussing past injustices with parents should
not be to make them eat crow for what they have done. Crow tastes
terrible, and asking them to eat it is not likely to lead them toward a
conciliatory response. Despite their denials and counterattacks, most
parents who have been abusive covertly feel extremely guilty about
it already. Their worst fear is that their children hate them for it,
although they also may feel simultaneously that they deserve to be
hated and that their offspring are better off without them.

I coach patients on how to confront their parents about old hurts
that, through the lack of acknowledgement, continue to haunt the
parent-child relationship for both of them. Unfortunately, the word
confront has an adversarial connotation, as in *confrontation*. I have
not been able to find a good synonym that has a more conciliatory
sound. What is being confronted in the sense that I am using the
word here is not a person per se, but the unfinished business
between two people.

The object of confronting parents about dysfunctional family
behavior should be to get them to stop behaving in ways that continue to reinforce an individual's self-destructive acting out, and
to reconcile with them. Even after successful metacommunication,
the person who has confronted the problem may still not want to
get really close to particular family members. He or she should,
however, feel comfortable enough being around them so as not
to constantly walk on eggshells to avoid exploding with old
resentments.

FORGIVENESS

I do not tell my patients who were victims of abuse that they absolutely must forgive their parents for past misdeeds in order to move forward with their lives. Fortunately, when metacommunication works well, forgiveness is a natural byproduct. It seldom fails to materialize. Of course, forgiving someone for something they have done is impossible if the person refuses to admit having done it in the first place. If parents, for example, continue to completely deny certain past behavior, the tension in the relationship with the formerly abused child will not ease for this reason.

Having said that, a successful confrontation does not require family members who have been abusive to acknowledge what happened explicitly. The acts do not have to be named or listed, the gory details of the abusive incidents do not need to be recapitulated, and the abuser does not have to go into an explosion of mea culpas. In fact, abject self-flagellation and falling down on one's knees begging forgiveness can be offensive maneuvers meant to lay a guilt trip on the confronter for ever having brought up an issue.

Indirect acknowledgement of past misdeeds and indirect apologies for them may not be as satisfying as direct ones, but once again, the object of such conversations should not be to make abusers suffer for their sins but to reconcile with them and improve current relationships. If the subject of a conversation between an abuser and an abusee is unspoken yet crystal clear to both parties from its context and implications, that is good enough.

For example, one of my patients was talking to her once physically abusive mother about how the patient's brother was treating his children. She and the mother discussed the physical discipline that was being employed by the brother. The patient stated that the brother should know better because of his own upbringing. This statement was obviously a less than subtle reference to the patient's own fate at the hands of her mother when she was a child. The patient then suddenly injected a question into the conversation. She said, "Mom, do you ever think about those old times?"

The mother replied, "Yes I do, and I regret a lot of them." The mother went on to explain that, after having given the matter much thought, she had come to the conclusion that when her children were small she always felt that she and they were a burden on their extended family. When the children made noise, she would become highly disturbed.

The specific acts of physical abuse that had resulted were never spoken of, but both of them knew very well exactly what the subject of the conversation was. The mother also never explicitly said, "I'm sorry for what I did." However, she expressed "regret" over some unnamed "times." Although it may not have sounded like one, this was an apology. The patient wisely did not ask her mother exactly what happened during the times she regretted. Their future conversations were a lot less tense from that point on.

A LAST WORD ON PARENTAL GUILT

If you are confronted with or learn something unpleasant about your performance as a parent, you can do one of three things. First, you can deny it and continue to lie to everyone, including yourself, but you will always know that it is true. Second, you can continually beat yourself up about it as if your shortcomings are written in stone and any harm you may have inflicted on your children is unforgivable and irreversible. The result of this course of self-damning action is continued guilt, which leads to more and more unpleasant feelings, which in turn lead to desperation, despair, and hopelessness.

Those choices will not only make you feel worse, but they also will not help your children feel any better about you, your relationship with them, or their childhood. It usually makes them feel even worse. A much better course of action is to forgive yourself for your human frailties, learn from your mistakes so that you do not repeat them, and talk openly with your offspring as best you know how about what had happened and why you felt and acted the way that you did. Your children really do, deep down, want to forgive you. Please let them.

No parent is perfect. Despite our best efforts, we all leave our children with some issues with which they have to struggle. Parents just have to be good enough, not flawless. If your children are still small, trying to protect them from all of life's naturally occurring adversity is counterproductive. Such efforts will weaken and impair your children, not make them stronger. What it takes to be a good enough parent is no mystery. It involves what have been termed the three L's: love, limit setting, and letting them go. If you have trouble providing all three of these things for your children because of your own upbringing, please get help. The transmission of dysfunctional family patterns from one generation to the next can be stopped.

A FINAL WORD

The mental health field is unfortunately filled with a lot of patent nonsense, as I have illustrated in this book. Thankfully, a lot of clinicians still do great work. The scientific knowledge base about brain functioning and social psychology has been increasing by leaps and bounds to the point where many old debates have been settled. Many new psychiatric drugs are more effective and have fewer side effects than older ones. Effective techniques for influencing the behavior of troubled people have also multiplied exponentially. Conflict resolution techniques and skills are readily available, so we all can learn to have more harmonious relationships with our loved ones. In this volume, I hope to have helped the reader to separate the wheat from the chaff.

My second goal in writing this book was to help the reader understand some mysterious aspects of human nature and to point out the hidden altruism that is often behind problematic behavior. I also have raised issues that point to a paradox created by misplaced altruism. By attempting to shield children from all adversity, parents can inadvertently lead their children to sacrifice themselves and become self-destructive based on their misinterpreted understanding of the parents' needs. Parents who, because of a sense that their adult children are better off without them, push their children away through cruel or unpleasant behavior not only punish themselves but also do the children no favors.

The quest for interpersonal understanding and reconciliation is a magnificent undertaking. I highly recommend it.

References

INTRODUCTION

1. Eisenberg, L. (1986). Mindlessness and brainlessness in psychiatry. *British Journal of Psychiatry, 148*, 497–508.
2. American Psychiatric Association. (1994). *Diagnostic and Statistical Manual of Mental Disorders* (4th ed.). Washington, DC: American Psychiatric Association.
3. Allen, D. (1988). *A Family Systems Approach to Individual Psychotherapy* (originally titled *Unifying Individual and Family Therapies*). Northvale, NJ: Jason Aronson.
4. Allen, D. (1991). *Deciphering Motivation in Psychotherapy*. New York: Plenum.
5. Allen, D. (2003). *Psychotherapy with Borderline Patients: An Integrated Approach*. Mahweh, NJ: Lawrence Erlbaum.

CHAPTER 1: THE BRAINLESSNESS-MINDLESSNESS PENDULUM

1. Kennedy, F. (1942). The problem of social control of the congenital defective. *American Journal of Psychiatry, 99*, 13–16.
2. Kanner, L. (1942). Exoneration of the feebleminded. *American Journal of Psychiatry, 99*, 17–22.
3. Editors. (1942). Euthanasia. Editorial, *American Journal of Psychiatry, 99*, 141–143.
4. Eisenberg, L. (1986). Mindlessness and brainlessness in psychiatry. *British Journal of Psychiatry, 148*, 497–508.
5. Herrnstein, R. J., & Murray, C. (1996). *Bell Curve: Intelligence and Class Structure in American Life*. New York: Free Press.

CHAPTER 2: DON'T BLAME US

1. Feshbach, S., & Singer, R. D. (1970). *Television and Aggression*. San Francisco: Jossey-Bass.

CHAPTER 3: THE "ABUSE EXCUSE" REVISITED

1. Flaherty, E. G., Sege, R. D., Griffith, J., et al. (2008). From suspicion of physical child abuse to reporting: Primary care clinician decision-making. *Pediatrics, 122*(3), 611–619.
2. Whitfield, C. L. (1987). *Healing the Child Within: Discovery and Recovery for Adult Children of Dysfunctional Families*. Deerfield Beach, FL: Health Communications, Inc.
3. Allen, D. (1988). *A Family Systems Approach to Individual Psychotherapy* (originally titled *Unifying Individual and Family Therapies*). Northvale, NJ: Jason Aronson.
4. Herman, J. L., & Schatzow, E. (1987). Recovery and verification of memories of childhood sexual trauma. *Psychoanalytic Psychology, 4*(1), 1–14.
5. Robins, L. N., Schoenberg, S. P., Holmes, S. J., et al. (1985). Early home environment and retrospective recall: A test for concordance between siblings with and without psychiatric disorders. *American Journal of Orthopsychiatry, 55*(1), 27–41.
6. Loftus, E. F., & Ketcham, K. (1994). *The Myth of Repressed Memory*. New York: St. Martin's Press.
7. Soloman, R. L., & Postman, L. (1952). Frequency of usage as a determinant of recognition thresholds for words. *Journal of Experimental Psychology, 43*, 195–202.
8. Williams, L. M. (1994). Recall of childhood trauma: A prospective study of women's memory of child sexual abuse. *Journal of Consulting and Clinical Psychology, 62*(6), 1167–1176.
9. Rinne, T., de Kloet, D. R., Wouters, L., et al. (2002). Hyperresponsiveness of hypothalamic-pituitary-adrenal axis to combined dexamethasone/corticotropin-releasing hormone challenge in female borderline personality disorder subjects with a history of sustained childhood abuse. *Biological Psychiatry, 52*, 1102–1112.

CHAPTER 4: IT'S A DISEASE! PSYCHIATRY AND PSYCHOLOGY SELL OUT

1. Mojtabai, R., & Olfson, M. (2008). National trends in psychotherapy by office-based psychiatrists. *Archives of General Psychiatry, 65*(8), 962–970.
2. Angell, M. (2004). *The Truth about the Drug Companies*. New York: Random House.
3. McManamy, J. (2002). Fanfare for the common salt. *McMan's Depression and Bipolar Weekly, 4*(26), August 2. http://mcmanweb.com/newsletter1.htm.
4. Posternak, M. A., & Mueller, T. I. (2001). Assessing the risks and benefits of benzodiazepines for anxiety disorders in patients with a history of substance abuse or dependence. *American Journal of Addictions, 10*, 48–68.

5. Maguire, E. A., Gadian, D. G., Johnsrude, I. S., et al. (2000). Navigation related structural change in the hippocampi of taxi drivers. *Proceedings of the National Academy of Science USA, 97,* 4398–4403.
6. Schwenkreis, P., El Tom, S., Ragert, P., et al. (2007). Assessment of sensorimotor cortical representations asymmetries and motor skills in violin players. *European Journal of Neuroscience, 26*(11), 3291–3302.

CHAPTER 5: THE HEREDITY VERSUS ENVIRONMENT DEBATE REVISITED: WHAT THE SCIENCE ACTUALLY SAYS

1. Chompsky, N. (1980). *Rules and Representations.* New York: Columbia University Press.
2. Cook, T. D., & Campbell, D. T. (1979). *Quasi-Experimentation: Design and Analysis Issues for Field Settings.* Boston: Houghton Mifflin.
3. Fonagy, P., Gergely, G., Jurist, E. L., & Target, M. (2002). *Affect Regulation, Mentalization, and the Development of the Self.* New York: Other Press.
4. Vignerová, J., Brabec, M., & Bláha, P. (2005). Two centuries of growth among Czech children and youth. *Economics & Human Biology, 4*(2), 237–252.
5. Caspi, A., McLay, J., Moffitt, T. E., et al. (2002). Role of genotype in the cycle of violence in maltreated children. *Science, 297,* 851–854.
6. Ducci, F. E., Hodgkinson, C., Xu, K., et al. (2008). Interaction between a functional MAOA locus and childhood sexual abuse predicts alcoholism and antisocial personality disorder in adult women. *Molecular Psychiatry, 13*(3), 334–347.
7. Brothers, L. (1997). *Friday's Footprint.* New York: Oxford University Press.
8. Medina, J. (1998). Long-term memory lane. *Psychiatric Times,* October, 21–23.
9. Siegel, D. (1999). *The Developing Mind: Toward a Neurobiology of Interpersonal Experience.* New York: Guilford Press.
10. Brothers, L. (1989). A biological perspective on empathy. *American Journal of Psychiatry, 146*(1), 10–19.
11. Brothers, L. (1997). *Friday's Footprint.* New York: Oxford University Press.
12. Lott, D. A. (2003). Unlearning fear: Calcium channel blockers and the process of extinction. *Psychiatric Times,* May, 9–12.
13. Asch, S. E. (1956). Studies of independence and conformity: A minority of one against a unanimous majority. *Psychological Monographs, 70*(9), 416.
14. Milgram, S. (1963). Behavioral study of obedience. *Journal of Abnormal and Social Psychology, 67,* 371–378.

CHAPTER 6: EVIDENCE-BASED IGNORANCE

1. Institute of Medicine. (2000). *To Err Is Human: Building a Safer Health System.* Washington, DC: National Academies Press.
2. Luborsky, L., & Crits-Cristoph, P. (1990). *Understanding Transference: The Core Conflictual Relationship Theme Method.* New York: Basic Books.
3. Smith, G. C., & Pell, J. P. (2004). Parachute use to prevent death and major trauma related to gravitational challenge: Systematic review of [randomized] controlled trials. *Journal of the International Association of Physicians in AIDS Care: JIAPAC, 3*(4), 108–109.

4. Specter, M. (2001). Rethinking the brain: How the songs of canaries upset a fundamental principle of science. *The New Yorker,* July 21.

5. Osser, D. N. (2008). Cleaning up evidence-based psychopharmacology. *Psychopharm Review, 43*(3), 19–26.

6. Perlis, R. H., Perlis, C. S., Wu, Y., et al. (2005). Industry sponsorship and financial conflict of interest in the reporting of clinical trials in psychiatry. *American Journal of Psychiatry, 162*(10), 1957–1960.

7. Safer, D. J. (2002). Design and reporting modifications in industry-sponsored comparative psychopharmacology trials. *Journal of Nervous and Mental Diseases, 190*(9), 583–592.

8. Herres, S., Davis, J., Maino, K., et al. (2006). Why olanzapine beats risperidone, risperidone beats quetiapine, and quetiapine beats olanzapine: An exploratory analysis of head-to-head comparison of second generation antipsychotics. *American Journal of Psychiatry, 163*(2), 185–194.

9. Sachs, G. S., Nierenberg, A. A., Calabrese, J. R., et al. (2007). Effectiveness of adjunctive antidepressant treatment for bipolar depression. *New England Journal of Medicine, 356,* 1711–1722.

10. Rush, A. J., Trivedi, M. H., Wisniewski, S. R., et al. (2006). Acute and long term outcomes in depressed patients requiring one or several treatment steps: A STAR*D report. *American Journal of Psychiatry, 163*(11), 1905–1917.

11. Schneck, C. D., Miklowitz, D. G., & Allen, M. H. (2008). Dr. Schneck and colleagues reply (letter to the editor). *American Journal of Psychiatry, 165*(8), 1049.

12. Luborsky, L., Diguer, L., Seligman, D. A., et al. (1999). The researcher's own therapy allegiances: A "wild card" in comparisons of treatment efficacy. *Clinical Psychology: Science and Practice, 6,* 95–106.

13. Davison, G. C. (2006). President's column: An invitation to auseinandersetzen about the evidence-based practices in psychology task force report. *The Clinical Psychologist 59*(1–2), 1–4.

14. Jacobson, N. (1995). The overselling of therapy. *Family Therapy Networker* 19: 40–51.

CHAPTER 7: DIAGNONSENSE

1. Young, R. C., Biggs, J. T., Ziegler, V. E., & Meyer, D. A. (1978). A rating scale for mania: Reliability, validity and sensitivity. *British Journal of Psychiatry, 133,* 429–435.

2. Ruggero, C. J., Zimmerman, M., Chelminski, I., & Young, D. *Journal of Psychiatric Research, 44*(6), 405–408. Borderline personality disorder and the misdiagnosis of bipolar disorder. *Journal of Psychiatric Research.*

3. Merikangas, K. R., Akiskal, H. S., Angst, J., et al. (2007). Lifetime and 12-month prevalence of bipolar spectrum disorder in the National Comorbidity Survey replication. *Archives of General Psychiatry, 64*(5), 543–552.

4. Angell, M. (2004). *The Truth about the Drug Companies.* New York: Random House.

5. Barlas, S. (2008). Concern about psychotropic drugs and foster care. *Psychiatric Times,* July, 62.

6. Hammerness, P., Surman, C., & Sassi, R. (2008). ADHD in adults: Matching therapies with patients' needs. *Current Psychiatry, 7*(9), 50–62.

7. McCabe, S. E., Teeter, C. J., & Boyd, C. J. (2006). Medical use, illicit use, and diversion of prescription stimulant medication. *Journal of Psychoactive Drugs*, 38(1), 43–56.
8. Setlik, J., Bond, G. R., & Ho, M. (2009). Adolescent prescription ADHD medication abuse is rising along with prescriptions for these medications. *Pediatrics*, 124(3), 875–880.
9. Strohschein, L. A. (2007). Prevalence of methylphenidate use among Canadian children following parental divorce. *Canadian Medical Association Journal*, 176(12), 1711–1714.
10. Kollins, S., Greenhill, L., Swanson, J., et al. (2006). Rationale, design, and methods of the preschool ADHD treatment study (PATS). *Journal of the American Academy of Child and Adolescent Psychiatry*, 45, 1275–1283.

CHAPTER 8: SPINNING ON AXIS II: THE MYSTERY OF BORDERLINE PERSONALITY DISORDER

1. Nisbett, R., & Ross, L. (1980). *Human Inference: Strategies and Shortcomings of Social Judgment*. Englewood Cliffs, NJ: Prentice-Hall.
2. Donaldson, S., & Westerman, M. (1986). Development of children's understanding of ambivalence and causal theories of emotions. *Developmental Psychology*, 22(5), 655–662.
3. Selman, R. (1980). *The Growth of Interpersonal Understanding*. San Diego: Academic Press.
4. Harter, S. (1986). Cognitive-developmental processes in the integration of concepts about emotions and the self. *Social Cognition*, 4(2), 119–151.
5. Linehan, M. (1993). *Cognitive Behavioral Treatment of Borderline Personality Disorder*. New York: Guilford Press.
6. Benjamin, L. S. (1993). *Interpersonal Diagnosis and Treatment of Personality Disorders*. New York: Guilford Press.
7. Bowlby, J. (1988). Developmental psychiatry comes of age. *American Journal of Psychiatry*, 145, 1–10.
8. Masterson, J. (1981). *The Narcissistic and Borderline Disorders: An Integrated Developmental Approach*. New York: Brunner/Mazel.
9. Linehan, M. (1993). *Cognitive Behavioral Treatment of Borderline Personality Disorder*. New York: Guilford Press.
10. Watzlawick, P., Beavin, J., & Jackson, D. (1967). *Pragmatics of Human Communication*. New York: Norton.
11. Allen, D. (1991). *Deciphering Motivation in Psychotherapy*. New York: Plenum.
12. Lis, E., Greenfield, B., Henry, M., et al. (2007). Neuroimaging and genetics of borderline personality disorder: A review. *Journal of Psychiatry and Neuroscience*, 32(3), 162–173.
13. Haselton, M. G., & Nettle, D. (2006). The paranoid optimist: An integrative evolutionary model of cognitive biases. *Personality and Social Psychology Review*, 10(1), 47–66.
14. Allen, D. M., & Whitson, S. (2004). Avoiding patient distortions in psychotherapy with patients with borderline personality disorder. *Journal of Contemporary Psychotherapy*, 34(3), 211–229.

15. McGoldrick, M., & Gerson, R. (1985). *Genograms in Family Assessment.* New York: W.W. Norton.
16. Bryson, K., & Casper, L. M. (1999). *Co-resident Grandparents and Grandchildren.* Washington, DC: Current Population Reports, Special Studies, U.S. Department of Commerce, Economics and Statistics Administration, Bureau of the Census.

CHAPTER 9: A TOWER OF PSYCHOBABBLE? TODAY'S PSYCHOTHERAPY, THE IDEA OF MENTAL DEFECTIVENESS, AND FAMILY SYSTEMS ISSUES

1. Corsini, R. J., & Wedding, D. (eds.). (2007). *Current Psychotherapies* (8th ed.). Florence, KY: Brooks Cole.
2. Gabbard, G. (ed.). (2009). *Textbook of Psychotherapeutic Treatments.* Washington, DC: American Psychiatric Publishing.
3. Fromm, E. (1994). *Escape from Freedom.* New York: Holt Paperbacks. (Originally published 1941).

CHAPTER 10: INTEGRATION

1. Bowen, M. (1978). *Family Therapy in Clinical Practice.* New York: Jason Aronson.
2. Berne, E. (1964). *Games People Play.* New York: Grove Press.
3. Selvini-Palazzoli, M. S., Boscolo, L., Cecchin, G., & Prata, G. (1978). *Paradox and Counterparadox.* New York: Jason Aronson.
4. Benjamin, L. (1993). *Interpersonal Diagnosis and Treatment of Personality Disorders.* New York: Guilford Press.
5. Wile, D. (1981). *Couples Therapy: A Nontraditional Approach.* New York: Wiley.
6. Wilson, E. O. (1998). *Consilience: The Unity of Knowledge.* New York: Alfred A. Knopf.
7. American Psychiatric Association. (2000). Practice guideline for the treatment of patients with major depressive disorder (revision). *American Journal of Psychiatry, 157*(4), Supplement.
8. Bowen, M. (1978). *Family Therapy in Clinical Practice.* New York: Jason Aronson.
9. Benjamin, L. S. (2003). *Interpersonal Reconstructive Therapy.* New York: Guilford Press.
10. Wachtel, P. L. (2007). *Relational Theory and the Practice of Psychotherapy.* New York: Guilford Press.
11. Magnavita, J. J. (2005). *Personality-Guided Relational Psychotherapy.* Washington, DC: American Psychological Association.
12. Ryle, A. (2001). *Introduction to Cognitive-Analytic Therapy: Principles and Practice.* New York: Wiley.
13. Young, J. E., Klosko, J. S., & Weishaar, M. E. (2003). *Schema Therapy: A Practitioner's Guide.* New York: Guilford Press.

Index

About the Author

DAVID M. ALLEN, MD, is Professor of Psychiatry and the former Director of Psychiatric Residency Training at the University of Tennessee Health Science Center in Memphis, a position he held for sixteen years. Prior to that, he was in private practice in Southern California for thirteen years during the advent of managed care health insurance. Additionally, he has done research into personality disorders and is a psychotherapy theorist. He is the author of three books for psychotherapists: *A Family Systems Approach to Individual Psychotherapy, Deciphering Motivation in Psychotherapy,* and *Psychotherapy with Borderline Patients: An Integrated Approach,* as well as numerous journal articles and book chapters. He is associate editor for the *Journal of Psychotherapy Integration* and a former treasurer of the Association for Research in Personality Disorders.